Emergency Medicine: To The Point!
Written and Oral Board Review

Meena Pai, MD

Emergency Medicine: To The Point!
Written and Oral Board Review
Meena Pai, MD

ISBN-13:
978-0692804247

ISBN-10:
0692804242

Disclaimer: This book was written with as much accuracy as possible but please note that mistakes are definitely possible. The author disclaims any responsibility for errors or missing information within this book and also for any results or consequences secondary to the use of the information in this book. Readers are strongly advised to confirm all information in this book. The use of this information in a clinical or nonclinical setting is solely the professional responsibility of the practitioner. If any errors or omissions are seen, please provide feedback to meenapai@gmail.com for updates to be made on the website. Thank you very much and wishing you all the best.

About the Author: Dr. Pai is a Board Certified Emergency Medicine Physician who trained in New York City. Directly from High school, she attended a direct seven year Medical Program, Sophie Davis School of Biomedical Education. She completed her final two clinical years at SUNY Downstate and completed an Emergency Medicine Residency at New York Presbyterian Queens-Weill Cornell Medical College. She worked in Houston, Texas, with Team Health and Memorial Hermann, while living in Texas. She currently works as an Emergency Medicine Physician at various hospitals in New York City, Long Island and Upstate New York.

I dedicate this book to my warm, loving, selfless, hard-working parents and to all those in the medical field who love to learn, including students, residents, physicians, physicians assistants, nurse practitioners, nurses, etc.

Preface:

This book is intended for Medical Students, Residents, Attending Physicians, PA's, NP's, Students, Nurses and anyone else involved in the field of Emergency Medicine. The book will be thorough enough to contain the information listed on the next page, on each pathological process and chief complaint that is mentioned in the most important aspects of the current ABEM EM Model. The sources referenced, include the following textbooks: Rosen's Emergency Medicine and Tintinalli's Emergency Medicine. Also referenced is the most recent Model of Clinical Practice of Emergency Medicine. The First and Second Sections are intended to be used as a supplement to prepare for the <u>Emergency Medicine Written Board Exam</u> and learning Emergency Medicine in general. The Third Section is intended to be used as a supplement to prepare for the <u>Emergency Medicine Oral Boards</u> <u>(Note that the material in this section is also useful in reviewing for the written boards). The</u> <u>Fourth Section includes Major points to know in Emergency Medicine, including Quick</u> <u>pointers, some of which are in a Basic Question/Answer Format, in order to help you Recall</u> <u>Key concepts.</u> The last section is for <u>Questions to ask while searching of a job in the field of</u> <u>Emergency Medicine.</u> However, please do not use this book alone. Please supplement it with an authoritative text (ie. Rosen's, Tintinalli's, journal articles, etc) and Question Banks in order to have the strongest foundation of knowledge in the field of Emergency Medicine. This book is solely intended to serve as an adjunct to help understand and retain the information further. There is some room on some of the pages, in order for the learner to make notes while studying. Practice and Repetition is always a key process in learning. Good luck studying and Best wishes in all of your future endeavors. Wishing you all the best there is, always.

The General Format/Layout that is discussed in the book is as follows:

1. Pathophysiology/Pathology
2. Signs/Symptoms
3. Chief Complaints and Differential Diagnosis
4. Pertinent Questions to Ask in the History and pertinent positives and negatives, to aid in evaluation and documentation
5. Physical Exam Findings
6. Diagnostic Imaging/Studies/Labs
7. Treatment/Management/Medications
8. Consultation/Disposition/Follow up
9. Key Tips
10. Helpful Mnemonics
11. Conceptual Review Points and Facts to Aid in Recall (Some in Quick Q & A Format)

Sections:

I. Chief Complaints
   a) Differential Diagnoses
   b) Pertinent Questions (Pertinent Positives and Negatives)
   c) Possible Physical Exam findings
   d) Management

II. Pathologies by System (Cardiology, Gastrointestinal, Immunology, Rheumatology, Hematology/Oncology, Neurology, Dermatology, Orthopedics, Trauma, Musculoskeletal, Pediatrics (integrated per section), OBGYN, Renal, Genitourinary, Pulmonary, Infectious Diseases, Otolaryngology, Ophthalmology, Environment, Toxicology)

   a) Pathology
   b) Signs/Symptoms
   c) Diagnosis
   d) Treatment/Management/Medications
   e) Consultation/Disposition/Follow Up
   f) Additional Important Facts and Helpful Mnemonics

III. Oral Boards Review Section
   a) Chart to Use on Your Oral Boards
   b) Potential Board Review Scenarios

IV. Rapid Review! Quick Questions & Answers and a Review of Major Concepts to Know

V. Questions to Ask During Your Job Search

TABLE OF CONTENTS

I. <u>**Section I: Chief Complaints, Differential Diagnosis, Diagnosis and Management**</u>

II. Section II: Topics by System

III. Section III: Oral Board Review

Note:Topic review can also be used as a supplement/adjunct for written board review)

IV. Section IV: Rapid Review! Quick Questions & Answers and A Quick Review of Key Concepts to Know! Contains 226 Must Know Bullet Points!

V. Section V: Questions to Ask for Emergency Medicine Job Search

SECTION I: CHIEF COMPLAINTS AND DIFFERENTIAL DIAGNOSIS

I. Chief Complaints
    1. Pain and Differential Diagnoses to strongly consider

Headache (Differential Diagnosis)

Meningitis, Encephalitis, Carotid artery dissection, Vertebral Artery Dissection, Cerebral Venous Thrombosis (Cavernous Sinus Thrombosis), Sinusitis, Acute narrow angle glaucoma, Traumatic vs. Non-Traumatic Brain Hemorrhage (Subdural Hematoma, Epidural Hematoma, Subarachnoid Hemorrhage) Temporal Arteritis, Carbon Monoxide Poisoning, Pseudotumor Cerebri (Idiopathic Intracranial hypertension), Primary headaches (Migraine, Tension Headache, Cluster Headache), Rocky Mountain Spotted Fever, Acute Mountain Sickness, High Altitude Cerebral Edema, Hypertensive Encephalopathy, Metastases to Brain, CVA, Tumor, Abscess, Preeclampsia (Pregnant patients), Hypertensive Encephalopathy, Brain Abscess

Headache

(Pertinent Positives/Negatives/Findings)

Meningitis: Headache? Neck stiffness? Fever/Chills? Photophobia? Seizure? Nausea? Vomiting?

Encephalitis: Confusion? Headache? Seizure? Fever? AMS?

Carotid Artery Dissection/Vertebral Artery Dissection: Stroke symptoms (Dysarthria? Aphasia? Focal Weakness? Ataxia? Numbness? Neglect?) Headache, Neck pain, Facial pain? Tinnitus? Vertigo? Ataxia? Weakness? Nausea/Vomiting? Numbness? Diplopia? Dysphagia?

Cerebral Venous Thrombosis: Headache? Stroke? Seizure? Neuro symptoms?

Cavernous Sinus Thrombosis: Headache? Nausea? Vomiting, Fever? Eye pain? Proptosis? Ophthalmoplegia? Chemosis?

Sinusitis: Headache? Facial pain? Congestion?

Acute Narrow Angle Glaucoma: Headache? Eye pain? Nausea? Vomiting? Abdominal Pain? Vision loss?

Brain Hemorrhage: Sudden Headache? Neck pain? Nausea? Vomiting? Photophobia? Blurry vision? Trauma? Family History?

Temporal Arteritis: Elderly (>50). Headache? Visual loss? Fever? Lethargy? PMR (Polymyalgia Rheumatica: Jaw Claudication, Myalgias)?

Pseudotumor Cerebri (PTC): Headache? Eye pain? Double vision? Visual loss? N/V?

RMSF: Rash (Petechial)? Headache? Fever; Muscle aches? Note that all these do not have to present. Possible Exposure to area with Ticks?

AMS: Acute Mountain Sickness: Occurs at High Altitude. Headache? Dizziness? Weakness? Nausea? Vomiting?
HACE: High Altitude Cerebral Edema: Occurs at High Altitude. AMS? Ataxia?

Hypertensive Encephalopathy: Headache, Seizure, Nausea, Vomiting, Confusion/AMS, Blurry vision
Trigeminal Neuralgia: Pain that is very sharp on one side of the face

Primary Headaches: (Migraine, Cluster): Migraine: Visual changes, Light flashes, Photophobia, Phonophobia, Nausea, Vomiting. Cluster: Retro-orbital Pain, Rhinorrhea, Lacrimation, Miosis, Ptosis

CO Poisoning: Headache, Nausea, Vomiting, Syncope, Visual changes? Possible Chest Pain? Neurological symptoms? Family members or Pets also sick? Winter? Heating source?

Headache Physical Exam Findings/Management

Meningitis: Infants can present with: Refusal to feed. Lethargy. Irritability. In all others: Meningeal signs: Neck stiffness (Kernig's sign, Brudzinski's sign), Headache, AMS, Photophobia, Nausea, Vomiting, Possible Petechiae.
Management: Do a CT brain if concerned about a Mass Lesion: ie. Papilledema, Focal Neurological Deficits, Seizure; AMS, Hx of Neuro disease (Stroke), Immunocompromised (ie. HIV). Also do a CT if concern for a Bleed, Lumbar Puncture, CSF studies (Cell Count and Differential, Culture, Gram Stain, Glucose, Protein, Additional studies as needed (ie. Viral, Fungal). Management: Steroids. IV Antibiotics. Respiratory Isolation. Admit.

Encephalitis: CT brain, LP (Include all Cultures, etc). Treatment: If due to HSV, Acyclovir. If bacterial, antibiotics.

Carotid artery dissection: Partial Horner's syndrome is possible. CVA symptoms/signs (ie. Dysarthria, Aphasia, Weakness, Vision Loss, etc.) Diagnosis: CTA or MRI/MRA. Needs Neurosurgery consult Stat. Treatment: Anticoagulation (but Contraindicated if the dissection extends to the Intracerebral portion)

Vertebral Artery Dissection: Weakness, Ataxia, Dizziness. Diagnosis: CTA or MRI/MRA. Needs Neurosurgery Consult Stat. Treatment: Anticoagulation (but Contraindicated if it extends to the Intracerebral portion)

Cerebral Venous Thrombosis: Focal Neurological Deficits. Headache. Tx: Anticoagulation (if no contraindications)
Cavernous sinus thrombosis: Headache. Periorbital edema. Ptosis. Proptosis. Papilledema. Chemosis. CN 3, 4, or 6 Gaze palsy. Management is IV Antibiotics

Sinusitis: Sinus Tenderness on Palpation. Management: Antibiotics (ie Augmentin, unless contraindicated)

Acute Narrow Angle Glaucoma: Injected Conjunctiva, Increased Intraocular pressure (IOP). Hazy/cloudy cornea. Shallow Anterior Chamber. Nonreactive Mid Dilated Pupil. Stat Ophthalmology consult. Management: Topical Timolol, Topical Apraclonidine, Topical Pilocarpine. IV Acetazolamide. Mannitol.

Brain Hemorrhage: Stat Neurosurgery Consult

Temporal Arteritis: Tender scalp over Temporal region. May have Tender Temporal Artery (Dx: Often Elevated ESR (>50), Risk of delayed diagnosis is Blindness. Needs **Steroids** as soon as the diagnosis is suspected. Confirmative test is temporal artery biopsy (but don't wait on this to give steroids). Ophthalmology Consult. Admit.

Pseudotumor Cerebri (PTC): Papilledema, Eye exam, CT brain, Lumbar Puncture (Increased Opening Pressure is Present). Tx: LP relieves pressure and Acetazolamide

RMSF: Rash, Possible Neuro findings, Fever, Neck Stiffness, Photophobia, Arrhythmia, Nausea, Vomiting. May see Thrombocytopenia, Elevated LFT's, Hyponatremia. Tx: Doxycycline. Of note: Neurological symptoms and Renal involvement are indicative of a worse prognosis

AMS: Best treatment is Descent
HACE: Best treatment is Descent

CO poisoning: Tx is 100% O2 and in some cases Hyperbaric Chamber)
(Hyperbaric Chamber needed in the following patients with CO poisoning: (HBO for the following: Pregnant with COHb >15%, COHb level >25% in anyone, Focal Neurological Deficit, Neuro Symptoms (ie Altered mental status, Seizure, Syncope), Myocardial Infarction

Eye Pain Differential Diagnosis

Acute Narrow Angle Glaucoma, Trauma vs. Nontrauma, Corneal Abrasion, Corneal Ulcer, Uveitis, Globe Rupture, Chalazion, Hordeolum (Stye), Keratitis, Retinal Detachment, Preseptal (Periorbital) Cellulitis, Postseptal (Orbital) Cellulitis, Eye Foreign Body, Blepharitis, Chemical Burn, Endophthalmitis. Retrobulbar Hematoma, Hyphema

Eye Pain Pertinent Positives/Negatives and Detailed Eye Exam

Eye Pain? Redness? Swelling? Vision Loss? Blurry Vision? Discharge? Photophobia? Tearing? Nausea? Vomiting? Headache? Neck pain? Abdominal pain? Trauma? Foreign Body sensation? Foreign Body? Curtain coming down Eye sensation? Floaters? History of Eye Surgeries?

Physical exam findings: External Inspection, Visual acuity, Slit Lamp findings, Fundoscopic exam, Pupil Reactivity and Size? EOM testing. Tonopen to Measure IOP (Only if it's Not Contraindicated: **Contraindicated** in Globe Rupture), Lid Eversion for suspected Foreign Body, Fluorescein Testing for Suspected Corneal Abrasion

Tenderness? Edema? Erythema? Proptosis? Ophthalmoplegia? Hazy/Cloudy Cornea? Subconjunctival Hemorrhage? Injected Cornea?

Eye Pain Management

Orbital Cellulitis: Postseptal Cellulitis: Infection involves the Orbit itself. Eyelid Edema and Erythema, Proptosis, Ophthalmoplegia, Chemosis, Possible Fever. Diagnosis is CT Orbit with Contrast. Treatment is IV Antibiotics (ie Unasyn). Stat Ophthalmology Consult is needed.

Periorbital Cellulitis: Preseptal Cellulitis: Anterior to the orbital septum. No orbital involvement. Eyelid Erythema and Edema. Diagnosis: CT Orbit with Contrast. Management: Antibiotics

Acute Narrow Angle Glaucoma: Headache, Pain in the Eye, Abdominal pain, Nausea, Vomiting. Cloudy Cornea, Mid-Dilated Pupil, Injected Conjunctiva, IOP is elevated. Stat Ophthalmology Consult. Treatment is Topical Beta Blocker (Timolol), Topical Alpha Agonist (Apraclonidine), Carbonic Anhydrase Inhibitor (Acetazolamide) IV, Mannitol IV, Check IOP every one hour, Topical Pilocarpine and Stat Ophthalmology Consult in the ER and Admission

Corneal Abrasion: Tear of the Cornea. Painful, Tearing, FB sensation, Photophobia, Eye scratched often times. Needs Fluorescein testing. Give Antibiotic Eyedrops and Ophthalmology follow up immediately if moderate to large in size. What is **Contraindicated?** Never patch eye.

Corneal Ulcer: Often in contact lens users. Symptoms similar to above. See a white stain on the cornea that is visualized with fluroscein. Needs stat Ophthalmology consultation in the ER immediately and antibiotics. What is **Contraindicated?** Never patch eye.

Globe rupture: Trauma. + Siedel's sign. Cover the Eye with a Shield. Consult Ophthalmology Stat. Give Antibiotics. What is **Contraindicated** in these patients? Do **Not** use a tonopen

Chalazion: Erythematous, Edematous Nodule on Eyelid. Management is Warm Compress and Ophthalmology follow up

Hordeolum: Stye: Needs Topical Antibiotics and Warm Compresses

Retinal Detachment: Retina is No longer attached properly to its epithelium. Needs Stat Ophthalmology Consultation. Presents with Floaters and that can progress to Visual loss. Can be seen on Orbital Ultrasound. Needs Surgical Repair by Ophthalmologist. Admit.

Retrobulbar Hematoma: Needs Stat Ophthalmology Consult and a Lateral Canthotomy

Chest Pain

Myocardial infarction (STEMI, NSTEMI), Unstable angina, Stable Angina, Aortic Dissection, Boerhaave's (Esophageal Rupture), Pericarditis, Pericardial Effusion/Cardiac Tamponade, Pneumothorax, Pulmonary Embolism, Trauma vs Non-trauma, Cocaine Induced Chest pain (can be a STEMI, etc), Pneumonia, Esophagitis, Musculoskeletal, GERD

Chest Pain Questions to Ask:

Location, Quality, Sudden or Gradual, Intermittent/Constant, Radiation, Onset, Duration, Alleviating and Exacerbating factors, Positional, Precipitating Events, at Rest or with Exertion or Both? Prior Episodes? How Different? Fever, Cough, Trauma, Shortness of Breath, Sweating, Nausea, Vomiting (Before or After Onset of Chest Pain), Weakness, Numbness/Tingling, Syncope, Abdominal Pain, Back Pain, Leg Pain/Swelling, Headache, Neck Pain, Prior Episodes, PMH, etc. PE risk factors (Prolonged Immobilization like Surgeries, Long Plane or Car Rides; Hx of Malignancy, Hx of PE or DVT, Family History of Thrombophilias, OCP use, Smoking, Pregnancy, Obesity). Ask Family History (Premature Heart Disease, Early/Sudden Death, Heart Disease), Alcohol use (When Last? Prior to Chest pain? Vomiting and then Chest pain or Vice Versa?) Drug use? (Cocaine use? When Last?) Always Err on the side of Admission/Keeping patients for Observation who have Risk Factors for Cardiac disease. Consult Cardiologist (or appropriate specialist, depending on the Diagnosis)

Chest Pain Management Part I

STEMI —> STAT Cath Lab Activation for PCI
NSTEMI —> Admit to Cardiology (Aspirin, Anticoagulation)
Pulmonary Embolism —> Anticoagulation (ie LMWH (Lovenox) or Heparin)
Pneumonia —> IV Antibiotics and usually Admit
Tension Pneumothorax —> Needle Decompression and then Chest Tube
Pneumothorax —> Chest Tube
Cardiac Tamponade —> Pericardiocentesis
Cocaine induced chest pain —> Aspirin, Benzodiazepines, Nitroglycerin, Oxygen (What's contraindicated? Beta blockers (don't ever give this in cocaine patients with chest pain because it causes uninhibited alpha adrenergic activity)
Aortic dissection: Tear in Aorta creating a False Lumen. If hypertensive, give Beta Blocker first (ie Esmolol) and then Vasodilator (Nitroprusside). Beta Blocker first in Aortic Dissection HTN to Prevent Reflex Tachycardia. Vascular Surgeon Consult Stat. Reminder: How can Aortic Dissection present? Severe Chest Pain, Back Pain, Neurological Deficits, Weakness, Dizziness, Ataxia, Syncope, Pulse Deficits/Differential, Paresthesias, Dysarthria, Aphasia, Aortic Regurgitation Diastolic Murmur. Reminder: It can present with CVA (neurological deficits) or MI, Cardiac Tamponade, Hemothorax, Aortic Insufficiency, Horner's Syndrome, Hoarse voice/Voice change, Mesenteric Ischemia, Renal failure. Risk factors: HTN, Pregnancy, Men, Marfan's, Coarctation of Aorta, Elderly, Smokers, Cocaine users; CXR: Widened Mediastinum, Aortic Contour Abnormality, Pleural Effusion possible), CTA Chest and Abdomen with Contrast (if Stable). Cardiac Monitor, Oxygen, 2 large bore IV lines, Labs (CBC, CMP, PT/PTT, Lactate, D-Dimer, Cardiac Enzymes, Type and Cross), Urinalysis, EKG, CXR, CT scan Chest, Abdomen and Pelvis with IV contrast)
Always look out for Dissection in a STEMI patient! An Aortic Dissection can cause and present as a STEMI. In these (dissection) patients, **Never** administer thrombolytics nor anticoagulants nor plavix nor aspirin. They are all **Contraindicated!** Always use your better judgment and keep your differential for the most detrimental diagnoses in mind!
Stat Cardiothoracic surgery consult. If hypertensive, IV beta blocker first (ie. Esmolol or Labetalol) and then Nitroprusside.
Cardiothoracic Surgery for Surgical repair

Chest Pain Management Part II

Boerhaave's: Esophageal rupture (Full Thickness): Occurs s/p Vomiting with Force (ie Alcohol) or after a Procedure like an Endoscopy. Chest Pain, Possible Radiation to the Back, Abdominal Pain. Painful Swallowing. Difficulty Breathing. Fever. May have Crepitus on Neck, Chest Wall or Arm Exam. EKG, CXR (May see Subcutaneous Emphysema indicative of Pneumomediastinum), CT Chest/Neck with IV Contrast (if stable), IV fluids, IV Antibiotics, NPO, Pain meds, STAT Consult to Cardiothoracic Surgeon for OR repair

Back Pain
Differential Diagnosis

Ruptured Abdominal Aortic Aneurysm, Aortic Dissection, Ruptured Ectopic Pregnancy, Spinal Cord Compression (SCC), Cauda Equina Syndrome (CES), Epidural Abscess, Pancreatitis, Herniated Disc, Fracture, Pyelonephritis, Pulmonary Embolism, Retroperitoneal Hemorrhage, Trauma (ie Splenic Rupture), Osteomyelitis, Hematoma, Malignancy (Metastases), Renal Colic

Key Reminder: Did you know? Aortic Dissection can present with Chest Pain/Back Pain and even symptoms of a CVA (Weakness, Numbness, etc). It can present as an MI or CVA or Mesenteric Ischemia because of the blood supply that is getting occluded in the process. Always keep Aortic Dissection in your differential for Back Pain, Chest Pain, Neck Pain, Dysphagia, Hoarseness, Numbness/Tingling, Weakness. Pulse discrepancy possible between arms…and the list goes on!

Think of a Ruptured AAA when…
An Elderly Patient presents after a Syncopal Episode?
An Elderly Patient presents with Back Pain?
An Elderly Patient presents with Abdominal Pain?

Think of SCC, CES with Back Pain and Sensory
Deficits/Motor Deficits/Bowel or Bladder
habit changes!

Back Pain Questions to Ask/Physical:

Questions to ask: Location? Onset? Duration? Sudden onset? Radiation? Quality? Alleviating factors? Exacerbating Factors? Prior episodes? Trauma? Chest pain? Abdominal pain? Leg pain? Leg swelling? Fever/chills? Nausea? Vomiting? Weakness? Numbness/Tingling? Night sweats? Weight loss? Palpitations? Shortness of breath? Urinary changes? Bowel movement changes? (Retention/Incontinence)? Dysuria? Increased frequency? Hematuria? Syncope? Dysphagia? Hoarseness? Recent procedures on spine? LMP? Headache? Stiff neck? Able to ambulate? IVDA? PMH, Meds, Allergies, Social history (IVDA? Alcohol? when last?), Sexual history, Family history; Reminder: Do a thorough Abdominal exam, GU exam (chaperoned), Rectal exam (chaperoned), Neurological Exam, Heart exam, Back exam

Back Pain
Diagnosis and Management:

AAA Rupture: Abdominal pain. Stable (CT Abdomen/Pelvis to see if Ruptured AAA). In Unstable patients, an Ultrasound Abdomen can show the Presence of an AAA but **Not** whether/Not it's Ruptured. A Ruptured AAA Needs to go to the OR Stat with Surgery (Stat Surgery Consult) for Surgical Repair

Aortic Dissection: See Chest Pain Management Section

Ectopic Pregnancy: Abdominal pain, Vaginal bleeding/spotting in a Pregnant woman. Diagnosis: Pregnancy Test and Ultrasound and Management if Ruptured is Stat OBGYN Consult for the OR for Surgery.
In an Ectopic Pregnancy, If the patient is stable and meets all the criteria, consider Methotrexate with Stat OBGYN Consult. Either way, you need a Stat OBGYN Consult!

Spinal Cord Compression: Can present with Back pain and Sensory deficits/Motor deficits/Bowel or Bladder Habit Changes/Diminished Rectal Tone/Saddle Anesthesia. Needs Stat MRI and Stat Neurosurgery Consult. Steroids. If due to an infectious cause (ie. Epidural Abscess, needs IV Antibiotics)

Pancreatitis: Epigastric Pain radiating to the Back, N/V. Dx: Elevated Lipase. Management: IVF's (Get CT if concern for Complication of Pancreatitis)

Pyelonephritis: Infection of Kidney, N/V, Flank Pain. Dx: UA, Physical Exam: + CVA Tenderness. Management is IV Antibiotics

Abdominal Pain Differential Diagnosis:

Perforated Viscous, Hernia (Reducible, Irreducible (Incarcerated), Strangulated), Abdominal Aortic Aneurysm (Ruptured?), Aortic Dissection, Renal Colic, Appendicitis, Diverticulitis, Cholecystitis, Biliary Colic, Cholangitis, Choledocholithiasis, Pancreatitis, Mesenteric Ischemia, Ovarian torsion, Testicular torsion, Ectopic pregnancy, Small Bowel Obstruction (SBO), Fournier's Gangrene, Intussusception, Meckel's Diverticulum, Large Bowel Obstruction, Volvulus, Myocardial Infarction, Peptic Ulcer Disease, Esophagitis, Gastritis, Urolithiasis/Nephrolithiasis, Acute Narrow Angle Glaucoma, Epidydimitis, Hepatitis, UTI, Pyelonephritis, Pelvic Inflammatory Disease (PID), Tubo-Ovarian Abscess (TOA), Fitz-Hugh Curtis, Ovarian Cyst, Threatened Abortion, Incomplete Abortion, Inevitable Abortion, Crohn's disease, Ulcerative colitis, Pneumonia, DKA (diabetic ketoacidosis), Trauma vs. Non-trauma, Splenic Rupture, Strep Pharyngitis (children), Constipation, Pulmonary Embolism, Hereditary Angioedema, Sickle Cell Crisis, Herpes Zoster, Liver Abscess

Abdominal Pain Questions to Ask:

Abdominal Pain? Nausea? Vomiting? Back Pain? Chest Pain? Pain? Vaginal bleeding? Vaginal discharge? Pelvic pain? Fever? Chills? Dysuria? Increased frequency? Diarrhea? Constipation? Headache? Neck pain? Eye pain? Trauma? Pelvic pain? Testicular Pain? Weakness? Dizziness? Syncope? Recent Procedure/Surgery?

Location? RUQ? RLQ? Epigastric? LUQ? LLQ? Suprapubic? Generalized? Does it radiate anywhere? Where? (ie back?); Quality (dull, sharp, etc.); Precipitating events (ie fatty foods? foods?); Severity (scale 1 to 10); Duration? Onset? Sudden onset? Gradual onset? Constant? Intermittent? Alleviating factors? Exacerbating factors? Prior episodes? PMH, Past Surgical Hx, Social History, etc.

Do an Abdominal Examination and a Pelvic/Testicular Examination (with permission and supervised with a chaperone).

Send labs (CBC, CMP, Lipase, PT/PTT, Type and cross, EKG, Cardiac enzymes where applicable (ie. risk factors or age 40 plus), Blood Cultures where applicable), Urinalysis, Urine Culture, Imaging (CXR, CT, US depending on presentation and patient) and Pregnancy Test (Qual, Quant)!

Give Appropriate Pain medications, etc. (allergies…ask first!)

Always do Serial Abdominal Examinations to ensure patient is not worsening. Call Appropriate Consults (ie. Stat Surgery Consult if patient is peritoneal: rebound, guarding; Stat OBGYN Consult if concern for Ovarian Torsion, Stat Urology consult for Testicular Torsion)

Abdominal Pain:

Perforated Viscous: Physical Exam: Peritoneal Signs (Rebound, Guarding). Free Air on Upright CXR. Management: Stat Surgery Consult (Must go to OR immediately!) IV Antibiotics.

Hernia (Incarcerated, Strangulated): Dx: CT Abdomen/Pelvis: Needs Stat Surgical Consult for Operative Repair, IV Antibiotics.

Abdominal Aortic Aneurysm: See Back Pain Section.

Aortic Dissection: See Back Pain Section.

Renal Colic: CT Abdomen/Pelvis Noncontrast. Fluids. Pain Meds. Urology Consult or Follow Up

Appendicitis: Dx: CT Abdomen/Pelvis (Adults), In Pediatrics, Consider RLQ Ultrasound. Tx: IV Antibiotics and Stat Surgery Consult.

Diverticulitis: Dx: CT Abdomen/Pelvis. Tx: Antibiotics

Cholecystitis: Dx: RUQ US. Tx: IV Antibiotics and Stat Surgical Consult

Mesenteric Ischemia: "Pain out of Proportion", Lactate may be Elevated; CT scan. Tx: IV Antibiotics, Stat Surgery Consult and IR Consult.

Small bowel obstruction (SBO): CT or Xray Abdomen Flat and Erect: NPO, IVF's, NG tube, Surgery Consult

Fournier's Gangrene: Clinical Diagnosis, May see more with CT. Needs Stat Surgical Debridement and IV Antibiotics.

Intussusception: Ultrasound, Contrast Enema (Air Enema) (Stat Surgery and IR Consult)

Pelvic/Groin Pain Differential Diagnosis:

Fournier's Gangrene, Ovarian Torsion, Ectopic Pregnancy, Threatened Abortion, Abortion, Septic Abortion, PID, STD, UTI, Testicular Torsion vs. Epidydimitis (Male Testicular pain or Abdominal pain), Tubo-Ovarian Abscess, Renal Colic, Ovarian Cyst, Placenta Abruptio, Fibroid, Any Abdominal Etiology (ie Appendicitis), Endometriosis
Ask the same questions as listed in abdominal pain section

Pelvic/Groin Pain Diagnosis and Treatment:

Ovarian Torsion: Dx: Transvaginal Ultrasound with Doppler
Tx: Stat OBGYN Consult for OR
Ectopic Pregnancy: HCG Quant, Ultrasound. Must Consult OBGYN Stat
Must send patient to the OR if Unstable (Ruptured Ectopic)
If Stable and Fits all the criteria, Methotrexate
Septic Abortion: IV Antibiotics and Admit
PID: CMT, Adnexal Tenderness. Needs Antibiotics.
TOA: Dx: Ultrasound. Tx: IV Antibiotics and Admit.
Testicular Torsion: Testicular US. Tx: Urology Consult Stat for OR
Fournier's Gangrene: Needs Stat Surgery Consultation for
Surgical Debridement and Needs IV Antibiotics

Altered Mental Status Differential Diagnosis

Hypoglycemia, Toxins (ie. Alcohol, Medication/Drug overdose or Drug withdrawal), Infection (Meningitis, Encephalitis, Sepsis, Urosepsis, Pneumonia, etc.), Hypovolemia (ie. GI Bleeding, Dehydration), Trauma (ie. CNS Bleed: SAH, Epidural, Subdural, ICH), Hypoxia, Uremia, Thyroid (Thyroid storm vs. Myxedema Coma), Seizure, MI, CHF, CVA, Brain Tumor, Brain Abscess, Electrolyte abnormalities (ie. Hypernatremia, Hypercalcemia, etc.), Hypertensive Encephalopathy, ruptured AAA, aortic dissection, ruptured ectopic pregnancy, Hepatic Encephalopathy, Neuroleptic Malignant Syndrome (NMS), Serotonin Syndrome, Adrenal Crisis, Medication interactions, Uremia, Altitude Sickness (AMS, HACE), Heat Stroke, Hypothermia

Altered Mental Status Mnemonic:

The Mnemonic for Altered Mental Status is...

OURS COME NEAT

Opiates, Uremia (Renal insufficiency), Sepsis, Stroke, Seizure, Serotonin Syndrome, CVA, CO poisoning, Cardiac (MI, Dysrhythmias), Overdose (Drug, Alcohol), Meningitis, Encephalitis, Encephalopathy (Hepatic), Encephalopathy (Hypertensive), Endocrine (Thyroid Storm, Myxedema Coma, Adrenal Crisis), Electrolytes (Hypoglycemia, Hyperglycemia, Hyperkalemia, Hypercalcemia, Hypocalcemia, Hyponatremia, Hypernatremia, etc.), NMS, Eclampsia, Alcohol, Altitude Sickness (Acute Mountain Sickness, HACE), Toxins, Tamponade, TTP, Temperature (Heat Stroke, Hypothermia), Tumor, Thyroid storm, Trauma

Altered Mental Status

Reversible: Hypoglycemia (Check Fingerstick glucose: if Hypoglycemic, give D50), Narcotic overdose (if pinpoint pupils and suspected narcotic OD, give narcan); if Hypoxic, give O2. If patient shows no improvement in mental status despite these measures and cannot maintain airway (ie. GCS <8 and no gag reflex), intubation should be strongly considered.

TIPS!

Tip: Always get a urine pregnancy test on a woman who is of child bearing age (even if they deny sexual activity)!
Tip: Always get a fingerstick glucose level in a patient with altered mental status, early in the evaluation!
Tip: consider infection/toxin, overdose, withdrawal/hypoglycemia/hyperglycemia/electrolyte abnormality/trauma/CNS bleed/GI bleed/hemorrhage/hypovolemia/shock/stroke/MI/polypharmacy/endocrine (thyroid, adrenal)/pregnancy/etc. and order tests reflecting the most likely etiologies - start with vitals and fingerstick glucose.
Tip: There are more than 4 vital signs in the critical patient! These are: BP, HR, 02 sat, RR, Temperature, Fingerstick glucose
Tip: Altered mental status has a huge differential diagnosis - divide it into categories (toxins/overdose/withdrawal, infection/sepsis, endocrine, neurological, traumatic, hemorrhage, hypovolemia, shock, cardiac/vascular, electrolytes, etc.)
AMS Mnemonic: **OURS COME NEAT**

Constipation

SBO, Ileus, Volvulus, LBO, Spinal Cord Compression, Epidural Abscess, Cauda Equina Syndrome, Electrolyte Abnormality (ie. Hypercalcemia), Medication use (ie. Opioid), Hirschsprung's

Abdominal pain? Nausea? Vomiting? Fever? Last BM? History of surgeries? Back pain? Leg Pain? Numbness/Weakness/Tingling? Medications? Changes in Bowel/Bladder Habits?

If SCC is a concern, a thorough neurological exam and a rectal exam are needed! check for saddle anesthesia too!

Cough

Pneumonia, Pulmonary Embolism, Pleural Effusion, Congestive Heart Failure, COPD, Pertussis, Foreign Body, URI, Bronchitis, Asthma, Allergic reaction, Medications (ACEI's), Lung cancer, GERD, Sinusitis, Croup, TB, URI, Bronchiolitis, Malignancy

Chest pain? Dyspnea? Fever? Nausea? Vomiting? Leg pain? Leg swelling? Fever? Weight loss? Night sweats?

Smoker?

Crying/fussiness

Hair tourniquet, Torsion, Infection/Sepsis/Meningitis/UTI/Pneumonia/Bronchiolitis; Intracranial Hemorrhage, CHF, Cardiac issues (Aneurysm, MI, Dysrhythmias), Abdominal problems (SBO, Intussusception, Pyloric Stenosis, Volvulus, Appendicitis, Hernia, etc.), Trauma, Electrolyte abnormality, Foreign Body, Abuse, Corneal Abrasion

Cyanosis

Medications, High altitude, Cold environment, Pulmonary embolism, Shock, Congenital heart disease, Methemoglobinemia, Peripheral vascular disease, Pulmonary Disease, Cardiac Disease

Hemoptysis

Cancer (lung ca), CHF, Pulmonary Embolism, Thoracic Aortic aneurysm, Bronchitis, Bronchiectasis, Pneumonia, Mitral stenosis, Anticoagulants and other medications that can cause bleeding; Lung Abscess, Procedure (ie Bronchoscopy), Coagulopathy, Autoimmune d/o (is. Goodpasture's), Tuberculosis, Infectious, Trauma, Endocarditis, Lupus, fistula, AVM

Large amounts of hemoptysis (Massive is >600 mL blood in a 24 hr period) is often due to the pulmonary or *bronchial arteries*. Bronchial more likely to lead to heavy hemoptysis (life threatening); first priority: Airway! assess need for immediate airway intervention; some patients need intubation if massive hemoptysis; if patient is stable and if able to provide a history, ask how much, what color; history, etc. CBC, CMP, Type and cross, PT/PTT, CXR, UA, EKG, CT chest; Consult thoracic surgery, pulmonary (intensivist); bronchoscopy; possible angiography; In a stable patient who is at high risk of a concerning cause of hemoptysis, err on the side of caution and do the CT chest as well.

Dizziness

Vertigo vs. Lightheadedness, Acute vs Chronic, Associated symptoms

Differential Diagnosis: Carotid artery dissection, Malignancy, CVA (Stroke), Dysrhythmia, Multiple sclerosis, BPPV, Meniere's, Labyrinthitis, Acoustic Neuroma, MI, Dehydration, Infectious (Sepsis, UTI, etc.), Toxins, GI Bleed, Hypoglycemia, Electrolyte abnormalities (ie. Hyponatremia, Hypocalcemia, Hypokalemia etc)

Lightheaded or Room Spinning Sensation? Affected by head movement? How?
Sudden onset? Gradual Onset?
Associated symptoms? Headache? Neck pain? Visual changes? Weakness?
Ataxia? Nausea? Vomiting? Tinnitus? Hearing Loss? Ear pain?
Chest pain? Dyspnea? Abdominal pain? Back pain?
Fever/chills? Syncope? Urinary Symptoms? Altered mental Status? Bleeding (dark or bloody stools?) Trauma?
Alleviating factors? Exacerbating factors?

Dyspnea

Pulmonary Embolism, Myocardial Infarction/ACS, Congestive Heart Failure (CHF), Heart Failure, Chronic Obstructive Pulmonary Disease (COPD), Asthma, Pneumonia, Pneumothorax, Pleural Effusion, Anaphylaxis, Pericarditis, Cardiac Tamponade, Arrhythmia, Cardiomyopathy, Symptomatic Anemia, Diaphragmatic rupture, DKA, Tension Pneumothorax, CVA, Neuromuscular disorder (Myasthenia Gravis), Multiple Sclerosis, Guillain Barre Syndrome, Altitude Sickness (HAPE =High Altitude Pulmonary Edema), Fat Embolism, Amniotic Fluid Embolism, Allergic Reaction, Toxins, Carbon Monoxide Poisoning, Acute Chest Syndrome, Valvular Disorders, Flail Chest, Epiglottitis, Retropharyngeal Abscess, Foreign Body

Chest pain? Neck pain? Diaphoresis? Pain? Trouble Breathing? Trauma? Nausea/Vomiting? Fever? Cough? Leg pain? Leg swelling? unilateral? bilateral? Itchy skin? Rash/hives? Abdominal pain? Back pain? Weakness/Numbness/Tingling? Visual changes? Ataxia? Dysarthria? Precipitating events? Palpitations? DOE? PND? Orthopnea?Syncope? Sore Throat? PE risk factors: Immobilization (recent surgery? prolonged travel?); History Malignancy? History DVT or PE? History of Thrombophilia in family? OCP use? Obesity? CHF? MI? Pregnant? Smoker?

Nausea/vomiting

Abdominal issue (SBO, Hernia (Incarcerated, Strangulated), Mesenteric Ischemia, Ruptured AAA, Hepatitis, Pancreatitis, Appendicitis, Perforated viscous, Boerhaave's, Cholecystitis, Infectious, Intussusception, Pyloric stenosis, Cholangitis, Cardiac (MI), Diabetic Ketoacidosis (DKA), Pregnancy (Hyperemesis Gravidarum vs Early Pregnancy), PID, Ovarian Torsion, Testicular Torsion, Nephrolithiasis, Pyelonephritis, Vertigo, Carbon monoxide poisoning, Meningitis, Acute narrow angle glaucoma, Rhabdomyolysis, Anaphylaxis, Hypercalcemia, Poisoning (Mushroom, Tylenol, Digoxin, Aspirin, Methanol, Ethylene Glycol, Alcohol, etc.), SBP, Withdrawal (alcohol, opioid), Brain hemorrhage (SAH, epidural, subdural, etc.), Acute Renal Insufficiency, Heat illness (ie. Heat exhaustion, Heat stroke), High Altitude (AMS, HACE), Radiation, Snakebite, Pyloric Stenosis, Acute Renal Failure, Adrenal Crisis

Nausea/Vomiting Questions to Ask:

Abdominal pain? Back pain? Flank pain? Chest Pain? Neck pain? Dyspnea? Syncope? Palpitations? Weakness? Fever? Chills? Headache? Neck stiffness? Photophobia? Eye pain? Pregnant? Recent Travel - Where? PMH? Alcohol? Drugs? Trauma? Winter? Heating source? New Foods (ie mushrooms)? Sick contacts?

Sore Throat

Retropharyngeal abscess, Peritonsillar abscess, Epiglottitis, Ludwig Angina, Infectious, Pharyngitis (Strep, Viral), Gonorrhea, Chlamydia, Infectious Mononucleosis, HIV, Foreign Body, SJS

Stridor

Angioedema, Foreign body Aspiration, Retropharyngeal Abscess, Epiglottitis, Bacterial Tracheitis, Croup, Diptheria, Laryngomalacia

Syncope

Subarachnoid hemorrhage, Myocardial Infarction, Hypoglycemia, GI bleed, CNS Bleed, Seizure, Stroke, TIA, Ruptured AAA, Aortic Dissection, Pulmonary Embolism, Toxins (alcohol, drugs), CHF, AV Block, Carotid Artery Dissection, Anemia, Ruptured Ectopic Pregnancy, Brugada Syndrome, Prolonged QT syndrome, Hypertrophic Cardiomyopathy, WPW, Valvular heart disease (ie. Aortic Stenosis), Torsades, Bradycardia, Heart block, Medications, CVA/TIA, Vasovagal, any Dysrhythmia (V tach, V fib, etc.), Vertigo, Drop attack, Seizure, Temperature related (ie. Heat Stroke), Pericardial Effusion, Anemia

Headache? Neck pain? Nausea/Vomiting? Photophobia? Chest pain? Dyspnea? Fever? Abdominal Pain? Back Pain? Palpitations? Weakness/Numbness/Tingling? Leg Pain/Swelling? Precipitating events? Symptoms prior to passing out? What were they? What were you doing prior to passing out? Incontinence? Eye rolling? Postictal Confusion? Prior episodes? How long did syncope last? Has this occurred before? Family history of sudden cardiac death or Early Cardiac issues?

Management Ideas to Consider: Full Physical Exam, FSG, Labs (CBC, CMP, etc.), EKG, CXR, CT Head, Observation/Monitoring, etc.
Further studies (ie. CTA chest if PE is a concern and no contraindications)

Vaginal Bleeding

Differentiate whether the patient is Pregnant or Not (Must send a Beta-HCG Qualitative and Quantitative).

If Pregnant, Consider: Ectopic pregnancy, Abortion, Molar Pregnancy, Placenta Previa, Placentae Abruptio.

If Not pregnant, consider Fibroids, Dysfunctional Uterine bleeding, Period, Malignancy.

Either scenario, consider Infection.

Vaginal Bleeding/Spotting? How many Pads changed per Day? Pregnant? (Even if Patient states Not Pregnant, still need to order an Official Pregnancy test). Abdominal Pain? Back Pain? Nausea? Vomiting? Trauma? Syncope? Chest Pain? Dyspnea? Weakness? Dizziness/Lightheadedness?

Send Basic Labs (CBC, CMP, Coags, Type and Screen, etc). Look at CBC results of Hgb/Hct. Check Rh (In a pregnant patient who is Rh negative, give Rhogam if never received before). Send UA and Culture (In pregnant patients asymptomatic bacteriuria is possible).

Do a Pelvic exam (unless contraindicated - i.e. in the later trimesters, rule out a placenta previa first because a pelvic is contraindicated as it can cause massive bleeding).

Note: If Pregnant, Transvaginal Ultrasound with a BHCG level above 1500 should be demonstrative of an IUP.

If there is No IUP above this BHCG level, consider Ectopic Pregnancy in your differential. Ectopic Pregnancy Needs Stat OB Consult.

If the hormone level is lower than this, the differential includes: Early IUP vs Abortion vs. Ectopic pregnancy. Always consult OB. For patients who can go home (ie stable threatened abortion), they need follow up in 1 to 2 days, for a repeat US and HCG.

Any Unstable patient needs OB consult Stat and Admission

Any Confirmed Ectopic pregnancy needs Admission/OB consult Stat in the ER

Vertigo

Infection (labyrinthitis, etc.), BPPV, Meniere's, Toxins, Medications, Malignancy, Multiple sclerosis, Stroke, Seizure, Migraines, Tumor, Vestibular Neuronitis, Otitis Media

Visual Disturbances

Eye pain, Eye Swelling, Vision loss, Curtain Vision, Floaters, Burning, Blurry vision, Chemical entry to eye, Eye Foreign Body, Eye Trauma, Eye Discharge, Red Eye, Double Vision

Foreign Body, Corneal Abrasion, Corneal Ulcer, Temporal Arteritis, Acute Narrow Angle Glaucoma, CRAO, CRVO, Retinal Detachment, Hyphema, Uveitis, Chemical Exposure to Eye, CVA, Retrobulbar Hematoma, Globe Rupture, Vitreous Hemorrhage, Optic Neuritis, Conjunctivitis

Vaginal Discharge

STD, PID, Ectopic pregnancy, Abortion, TOA, Vaginitis, Pregnancy, Foreign Body, Infection

Wheezing

Asthma, COPD, Foreign body, Anaphylaxis, Bronchiolitis, Pulmonary embolus, Pulmonary Edema, Croup, Epiglottitis, Pneumonia

Paresthesias/Paralysis

CVA, TIA, Bell's palsy, Spinal Cord compression, Peripheral Neuropathy, Electrolyte disturbances, Dissection, GBS, Toxins, Endocrine disorders, Malignancy

Weakness

CVA, TIA, Aortic dissection, Myocardial Infarction, Hypoglycemia, Multiple Sclerosis, Transverse myelitis, Spinal Cord Compression, Cauda Equina Syndrome, Electrolyte disorders (Hyponatremia, Hypernatremia, Hypokalemia, Hyperkalemia, Hypocalcemia, Hypercalcemia), Sepsis, Infection (ie. Influenza, Pneumonia, Sepsis, etc.), Myxedema Coma/Hypothyroidism, Dermatomyositis, Polymyositis, Temporal Arteritis, SLE, Rheumatoid Arthritis, Anemia, Dehydration), Bleeding (GI Bleed), Endocrine (Thyroid, Adrenal, DM, etc.), Electrolyte abnormalities, Myocardial Infarction, Shock, Poisoning, Rhabdomyolysis, Multiple Sclerosis, ALS, Guillain Barre Syndrome, Myasthenia Gravis, Spinal Cord Compression, Botulism

Limp

SCFE, Septic arthritis, Legg Calve Perthes, Toxic (Transient) Synovitis, Fracture, Sprain, Developmental Hip Dysplasia, Malignancy, Sickle cell anemia, Osteomyelitis, Rheumatoid Arthritis, Rheumatic Fever, Concerning Abdominal Etiology (ie. Appendicitis), Any concerning etiology that causes pain could potentially cause a limp as well

Note: SCFE can have Referred pain (ie. Knee pain). May present with Hip Pain, Thigh Pain, Leg pain

Note: SCFE: Do Bilateral Hip X-rays. Needs Orthopedic Consult if SCFE is present for ORIF because if Acute and Not treated, it can lead to Avascular Necrosis!

Pediatric Limp: Usually use Ultrasound or X-ray (SCFE: Image both Hips with X-rays), depending on the concern

If Septic Arthritis: Arthrocentesis, Antibiotics, Orthopedic Consult and Admit!

Lower Extremity Pain Differential Diagnosis:

Acute Limb Ischemia, Arterial Dissection, Deep Venous Thrombosis (DVT), Cellulitis, Compartment Syndrome, Necrotizing Fasciitis, Septic Arthritis, Gout, Pseudogout, Trauma (Fracture/Dislocation/Ligament injury), Abscess

Hip fracture, Hip dislocation, Femur Fracture, Knee Dislocation, Knee Fracture, Tibial Plateau Fracture, Tibial fracture, Fibula fracture, Ankle fracture, Ankle dislocation

Foot: Lisfranc's fracture, Jones, Pseudojones, Calcaneal fracture and other fractures

Leg pain? Leg swelling? Fever? Where is the pain? Trauma?

Do a Full Neurovascular Exam, CV Exam, Extremity Exam

Pulses intact?

Unilaterally absent pulse: Consider Acute Limb Ischemia!

Compartment Syndrome: Pain? Paresthesia?

Cold? Pallor? Pulseless? Paralysis?

Lower Extremity Pain Diagnosis and Management:

Acute Limb Ischemia: Pain? Pallor? Pulseless? Paresthesias? Paralysis? Cold foot? Use Doppler to look for Pulse. Calculate ABI. Acute Limb Ischemia Needs Stat Vascular Surgery Consult. Admit.

Deep Venous Thrombosis (DVT): Dx: US Doppler. Tx: Anticoagulation

Compartment Syndrome: Dx: High Compartment Pressure. Tx: Fasciotomy

Necrotizing Fasciitis: Painful. Surgical Consult Stat. Needs Stat Surgical Debridement, IV Antibiotics

Septic Arthritis: Arthrocentesis. Orthopedic Consult Stat. IV Antibiotics.

Tip: Whenever a patient presents with any chief complaint, immediately think of all the differential diagnoses, starting with the most severe/lethal ones first - Remember to include pertinent positives and negatives in your notes to show yourself that you considered each diagnosis in your thorough evaluation of the patient.

Neck Pain Differential Diagnosis

Meningitis, Carotid Artery Dissection, Vertebral Artery Dissection, Subarachnoid Hemorrhage, Myocardial Infarction, Retropharyngeal Abscess, Peritonsillar Abscess, Ludwig Angina

Neck Pain Questions To Ask:

Neck pain? Headache? Photophobia? Numbness/Weakness/Tingling? Chest Pain? Nausea? Vomiting? Fever? Seizure? Facial pain? Trauma? Dyspnea? Syncope? Extremity Pain? Weakness? Numbness? Tingling? Dysarthria? Back Pain? Abdominal Pain? Dizziness/Lightheadedness? Fever? Sore Throat? Swelling? Drooling? Hoarseness?

Neck Pain Diagnosis and Management:

Meningitis: Dx: Lumbar Puncture. Tx: IV Steroids. IV Antibiotics.
Carotid Artery Dissection: See Headache Section
Vertebral Artery Dissection: See Headache Section
Subarachnoid Hemorrhage: Dx: CT, LP. Tx: Neurosurgery Consult, Nimodipine
Myocardial Infarction: STEMI needs PCI (See MI in Cardiology Section)
Retropharyngeal Abscess: Dx: Xray Neck Soft Tissue. Tx: IV Antibiotics, Stat ENT.
Peritonsillar Abscess: Tx: Needle Aspiration (ENT), Antibiotics
Ludwig Angina: Airway Management, Stat ENT, IV Antibiotics

Fever:

Abdominal (Cholecystitis, Appendicitis, UTI, etc. See Abdominal Pain section), Skin (Cellulitis, Abscess, Necrotizing Fasciitis), Fournier's Gangrene, Pneumonia, Pulmonary Embolus, ENT (Retropharyngeal abscess, Peritonsillar abscess, Strep Pharyngitis, Otitis Media, etc.), Neutropenic Fever, Meningitis, Infective Endocarditis, Heat exhaustion, Heat stroke, Neuroleptic Malignant Syndrome, Serotonin Syndrome, Malignant Hyperthermia, Thyroid Storm, Sepsis, Consider Infection from Catheter

Fever? Pain? Where? (Abdomen, Chest, Back, Neck, Head, Groin, Extremities, etc). Nausea? Vomiting? Cough? Sore Throat? Trouble Breathing? Precipitating Events? New Medications? Which ones? Leg Pain? Leg Swelling? Redness? Recent Procedures? PMH?

Key points:

Any baby 28 days old or less with a Fever gets a Full Septic Workup This includes a CBC, CMP, UA, Urine Culture, Blood cultures, CXR, CT Head if concern for Mass lesion, Lumbar puncture, CSF studies (Obtain informed consent for any procedures)

A Cancer Patient with a Fever and a Low WBC Count where ANC is <500 (Neutropenic fever): Reverse Isolation, Cultures, Antibiotics

If the source isn't obvious, do a thorough Physical examination (Skin, etc. especially on elderly patients) and also consider an Occult infection!

Recent Catheter Insertion...site infected?

Hematuria

Cancer (ie Bladder Ca), BPH, Infection (ie. UTI), Trauma,
Kidney stones, Autoimmune disorders (SLE, etc.),
Glomerulonephritis, Bleeding disorder (ie. Hemophilia), Sickle
Cell Anemia, Medications (ie. Anticoagulants), Trauma, AVM

Lymphadenopathy

Infectious, Malignant, Autoimmune disorders,
Inflammatory response, Medication induced

Ear

Ear pain, Ear Swelling, Ear Foreign Body, Ear Trauma, Hearing Loss, Ear Drainage/ Discharge/Bleed), Ear Redness, TM Rupture), Sore Throat? Otitis Media, Externa, FB, Malignant Otitis Externa (ie. DM, Elderly), Peritonsillar abscess

Ataxia

Brain tumor, CVA, Cerebellar issue, Toxin (ie Alcohol, Drugs), Medications, Electrolyte Disturbances, Multiple Sclerosis

Ascites

SBP, Biliary disease, Hepatitis, Liver failure, Cholangitis, Nephrotic Syndrome, Heart failure, Malignancy, Infection

Anuria

Renal failure, Obstruction, Toxins, Infection/Sepsis, Shock

Anxiety

Anxiety Differential: MI, PE, SAH, Dysrhythmias, Hyperthyroidism/Thyroid Storm, Toxins, Asthma, Airway Obstruction, Anaphylaxis, CHF, Pneumothorax, Anemia, Electrolyte abnormalities, Hypoglycemia, Pheochromocytoma

Try Not to Diagnose Anxiety in patients. This Diagnosis should be Avoided for the most part, as **more serious etiologies** can present with a patient feeling anxious. Let the vitals and tests that you conduct (Bloodwork and Imaging, depending on the scenario) lead the way.

Vital Signs:

Always keep your eyes open for abnormal vital signs and think of how to correct it, whether/not you should correct it (ie. the principle of cerebral autoregulation) and the reasoning behind it, along with a Differential Diagnosis!

Hypothermia *(Thyroid issue, Sepsis, Environment related, etc.)*
Hyperthermia *(Thyroid issue, Sepsis, Environment related, etc.)*
Bradycardia *(Medications, Electrolytes, Thyroid, Hypothermia, MI, CNS bleed, etc)*
Tachycardia *(Sepsis, Pulmonary Embolism, Bleed, ie. GI Bleed, Intracranial Bleed), Heart condition (ie. Arrhythmias), Anemia, Hyperthyroidism, etc.*
Tachypnea *(Electrolytes, Pulmonary, Cardiac, Medications, Thyroid, Sepsis, etc.)*
Hypoxia *(Pulmonary, Thyroid, High Altitude, Neuromuscular, Cardiac)*
Hypotension *(ie. Shock- Cardiogenic, Hypovolemic, Distributive, Neurogenic)*
Hypertension *(ie. Hypertensive Emergency -ie. Aortic Dissection, Hemorrhagic CNS Bleed, etc.)*

GASTROENTEROLOGY

STRUCTURAL

1. Hernias

a) Pathology - Protrusion of Contents of the Abdomen (ie Intestines) through a weakened portion of the abdomen or the section that it resides within

b) Signs/Symptoms - Abdominal pain, Nausea, Vomiting, Possible Fever. On Physical Exam, often Palpable in Abdomen/Groin, depending on the type

c) Types- Hernias can be Reducible (Able to Reduce), Irreducible (Incarcerated) or Strangulated (Blood supply cut off). Please note: An Emergent Surgical Consult is needed if the Hernia is Incarcerated (Irreducible) or Strangulated

d) Diagnosis - Physical Examination, CT scan Abdomen/Pelvis

e) Treatment/Management: NPO (No food by mouth), IV Fluids, IV Antibiotics (ie. if Strangulated), Emergency Surgery Consult and Admission (if either Strangulated or if Incarcerated). If reducible and asymptomatic, reduce the hernia and may discharge home with surgical follow up as soon as possible

f) Consultation/Disposition/Follow Up - Surgical Consult and Admission if Incarcerated or Strangulated Hernia or Persistent Pain/Nausea, Vomiting

g) Reminder: **Never** attempt to Reduce a Suspected Strangulated Hernia!

ESOPHAGUS

1. Boerhaave's

a) Pathology - Rupture of the Full thickness of Esophagus (Etiologies: Alcohol and Emesis, Vomiting with Force, Iatrogenic (Endoscopy), etc.)

b) Signs/Symptoms - Severe Chest Pain, Vomiting, Possible Back pain, Neck pain, Abdominal pain, Dyspnea. May find Subcutaneous Emphysema on exam. Hamman's Crunch (Due to Pneumomediastinum hear a Crunchy sound when listening to the heart)

c) Diagnosis - Clinical, CXR (May show a Pleural Effusion on the Left), CT Chest, Endoscopy

d) Treatment/Management/Medications - NPO, IVF's, IV Antibiotics, Stat Surgery Consult

e) Consultation/Disposition/Follow Up - Emergent Surgery Consult and Admission

f) Additional Facts - Consider in Patients who Vomited and then had Chest Pain. Consider in Alcoholics who Forcefully Vomited and then got Severe Chest Pain. Boerhaave's has a Very High Mortality Rate. Consider Esophageal Rupture in those with Recent Esophageal Procedures (ie. Endoscopy) as well.

g) Reminder: This Diagnosis is Often Missed, leading to very Adverse Consequences, so Always Keep this Diagnosis in Mind!

2. **Toxic Effects of Caustics**

a) Acids —> Causes Coagulation Necrosis

b) Alkalis —> Causes Liquefaction Necrosis. Usually Worse. Can cause Perforation and other Detrimental Consequences

c) Patients with Burns of the Esophagus can present with Vomiting, Abdominal pain, Painful/Difficulty swallowing, Airway Compromise secondary to Edema, Respiratory Distress. Ingestion of Caustics can lead to Burns, Bleeding and Perforation

d) Always secure ABC's first, Intubate early if needed (ie oral burns, unable to handle secretions, pooling of fluid in the mouth, etc.), IVF's, O2, labs, CXR, IV antibiotics, GI consult, possible endoscopy

3. **Mallory-Weiss syndrome:**

a) Pathology: Partial Tear of the Esophageal Wall. It can also be secondary to Valsalva maneuvers, Vomiting. Possibly Alcoholics. Often in those with Hiatal Hernias

b) Signs/Symptoms: Hematemesis usually after Forced Vomiting.

c) Diagnosis is Endoscopy

d) Management: Labs, Monitoring. Often times, it may resolve on its own. If it is Moderate/Severe, Needs Labwork (CBC, CMP, Coags, Type and Cross), IVF's, Possible PRBC's, Cardiac Monitoring, Admission and Possible Surgical intervention (ie. Embolization)

4. Esophageal Varices:

a) Pathology: Very Dangerous/Severe Bleeding that often occurs in those with Alcoholic Liver Disease, Cirrhosis. It is due to Increased Portal Pressure that subsequently causes dilation of veins in the esophagus

b) Signs/Symptoms: presents with Hematemesis/Melena or Coffee Ground Emesis

c) Diagnosis and Management: Needs Emergency GI Consult (Emergent Endoscopy) and IV Antibiotics, Octreotide. Endoscopy for Banding, Sclerotherapy. Possible TIPS

5. Esophageal Foreign Body

a) Children may present with Vomiting, Choking, Dysphagia, Odynophagia, Neck Pain, Sore Throat, Chest Pain, Drooling, Stridor and Not eating as symptoms. However, they may also be Asymptomatic. Any Symptomatic patient needs Admission and a Stat GI Consult for intervention (ie. Endoscopy). Mild symptoms needs Admission as well at least, for monitoring.

b) X-rays (A-P and Lateral views are needed)

c) On A-P view of X-ray you can see a Coin lodged in the Esophagus (Frontal view, Coronal view).

d) On the Lateral View, you can see a Coin lodged in the Trachea (Sagittal view).

d) You should always have a high degree of suspicion for this diagnosis (even if you don't see a foreign body on x-ray, as the object may be radiolucent).

e) When is an Emergency Endoscopy Necessary for a FB in the Esophagus? Respiratory distress, Pooling of secretions, Many foreign bodies, Pointy/ Sharp object, Elongated object, Airway compromise, Any Button Battery, Possible Perforation, Symptoms (GI bleeding, Abdominal pain, Nausea, Vomiting, Fever), If the Foreign Body has been in the patient for over a 12 hour period

f) A Button Battery Ingestion in the Esophagus is very dangerous! It can cause Perforation! It needs Emergent Endoscopy and IV Antibiotics

g) Needs Stat Consult to GI Stat

h) Esophageal Foreign Bodies are the Most Dangerous due to the Risk of Esophageal Perforation.

i) If a Foreign Body is deemed safe enough to watch, observe, do serial x-rays to ensure it it progressing, with GI follow up.

6. **Infectious Esophagitis** (Candida, Viruses (ie. CMV, HSV), Bacteria). Causes Painful Swallowing and Difficulty Swallowing. Diagnosis is Endoscopy. Management for Candida is Fluconazole. Treatment for Viral is the Appropriate Antiviral. For instance, the Treatment for HSV is Acyclovir. The Treatment for CMV is Gancyclovir. In this scenario, you can ask the patient if they want to be screened for HIV.

7. **Gastroesophageal Reflux (GERD):** Due to a Weak Lower Esophageal Sphincter that causes Reflux, Chest Burning Sensation. Be careful with this diagnosis! Always consider a Cardiac etiology first because they can manifest the same way! Management of GERD is PPI's (If No improvement, Endoscopy).
Reminder: Be very careful in your diagnosis because antacids can deceivingly help alleviate both Cardiac and GI induced Chest Pain! Don't miss an Atypical MI!

8. **Pill induced Esophagitis:** Causes may include: NSAIDs, Doxycycline, Potassium chloride, Clindamycin, Alendronate (bisphosphonate). Management: Stop the Medication. To try to avoid Pill induced Esophagitis, advise patients to take their medications with water.

9. **Tracheoesophageal Fistula:** Connection between the Trachea and the Esophagus. Can cause Coughing, Choking. Can cause Difficulty Breathing in the infant, during feedings due to this Connection. Needs Surgical Evaluation/ Management.

10. **Zenker's Diverticulum:** Pouch off the esophagus. Diagnosis is Barium Swallow, Endoscopy. Management is Surgical or Endoscopic removal

11. **Schatzki Ring, Esophageal Stricture:** Narrowing of the Esophagus that makes it Difficult to Swallow. Diagnosis is Barium Swallow or Endoscopy and Management is Endoscopy in order to Dilate the Stricture or Ring

12. **Esophageal Motor Disorders** (Can be caused by the following: CVA, Myasthenia Gravis, Scleroderma, Achalasia, Diffuse Esophageal Spasm (DES), Nutcracker Esophagus)

      a. **Scleroderma:** Multisystem disorder that affects the Skin, GI tract, Lung, Heart, Kidneys, Joints. It causes Fibrous tissue to replace normal tissue thereby, in the case of the Esophagus, making it difficulty to swallow

      b. **Achalasia:** The Lower Esophageal Sphincter Does Not Relax. Causes Difficulty/Painful Swallowing, Chest Pain. Diagnosis is Barium Swallow or Manometry or EGD. Treatment is either Surgical or Medications

      c. **DES:** Esophageal contractions. Diagnosis is Manometry. Treatment is either Surgical or Medications

LIVER

I. **Cirrhosis:**

    A. Pathology: Irreversible nodular degeneration of the liver which can be secondary to Alcohol, Toxins, Hepatitis, NASH, etc.

    B. Signs/Symptoms: Can manifest in a Multitude of ways, including Neurological (ie Hepatic Encephalopathy, Asterixis), GI (Nausea, Vomiting, Abdominal Pain, Esophageal Varices, GI Bleeding, Ascites), Electrolyte Abnormalities, Skin (Caput Medusae, Jaundice, Erythema), Hematological (Anemia, Coagulopathy), Edema, GU (Amenorrhea, Impotence)

    C. The Management depends on treating the underlying manifestation and the underlying precipitant

2. **Hepatic Encephalopathy:**

a) Pathology: This is due to the build up of waste products, like Ammonia, in Patients with Cirrhosis

b) Signs/Symptoms: AMS, Fatigue/Weakness, Asterixis

c) Diagnosis is Clinical but patient May have an Elevated Ammonia (Note: this is **not** diagnostic)

d) Treatment is Lactulose, Neomycin

3. Hepatorenal Failure:

a) New Onset Acute Renal Failure in Cirrhosis patients. Has a Very Bad Prognosis

b) Labs suggestive of Acute Renal Failure

c) Needs a Transplant

4. Abscess:

a) Purulent circumscribed collection in the Liver

b) May present with Abdominal pain, Fever, Nausea, Vomiting

c) Diagnosis: Labs (Elevated LFT's, etc). CT Abdomen/Pelvis.

d) Treatment is IV Antibiotics/Medications dependent on Infectious Etiology and Possible Drainage

5. **Hepatitis:** Hepatitis is due to Viruses, Bacteria, Other Bugs, Medications, Alcohol, Toxins, Mushroom (ie. Amanita Phalloides), etc. Hepatitis A and E are generally due to food sources that are contaminated. Hepatitis E can be dangerous in pregnant women. Hepatitis B, C, D are due to Blood, Saliva, Secretions, etc. A few sources are: Newborns with infected mothers, Sexual partners, IVDA, Needlesticks

GALLBLADDER, BILIARY TRACT

1. **Biliary Colic:**

   1. Pathology: Gallstone that is Temporarily Obstructing the Cystic Duct. Precipitant is often Fatty Foods

   2. Signs/Symptoms: RUQ pain, Nausea, Vomiting, Possible Radiation of Pain to the Shoulder

   3. Diagnosis: Clinical and Ultrasound of RUQ

   4. Management is Pain Medications and Surgical follow up if Patient is Stable and Pain resolves, PO tolerated well. Advise the Patient to Eliminate Fatty Foods from the Diet as they are often Precipitants to Biliary Colic

2. Cholecystitis:

1. Pathology: Inflammation of the Wall of the Gallbladder. Infection possible.

2. Signs/Symptoms: RUQ pain, Nausea, Vomiting, Fever/chills, Possible Radiation of the Pain to the Shoulder

3. Diagnosis: RUQ Ultrasound: Pericholecystic Fluid, Enlarged Gallbladder, Sonographic Murphy's sign, Gallbladder Wall Thickening

4. Management: NPO, IVF's, IV Antibiotics, Needs Stat Surgery Consult for Cholecystectomy

5. Helpful Points: Reminder! Not all Cholecystitis cases have to have Stones

   a. **Acalculous cholecystitis:** No stones present but the patient does have cholecystitis. Patients at risk of this are Elderly/History of Trauma/ Surgical Procedure/Diabetic/HIV/Immunocompromised/on TPN/Septic patients/Cardiac patients. Management: NPO, IVF's, IV Antibiotics, Stat Surgery Consult. Needs Stat Surgery because has a High Mortality!

   b. **Emphysematous Cholecystitis:** Occurs when Gas Forming Anaerobes cause Cholecystitis. Occurs in those with Cardiovascular Risk Factors, Diabetics. Dx is US or CT. Management: NPO, IVF's, IV Antibiotics, Stat Surgery Consult. This has a Very high mortality! Needs Stat Surgery

3. Choledocholithiasis:

1. Pathology: Stone in the Common Bile Duct

2. Signs/Symptoms: Fever, Chills, Abdominal Pain (ie. RUQ, Epigastric), Possible Nausea/Vomiting, Jaundice, Labs: Total Bilirubin Elevated, Alkaline Phosphatase Elevated, Increased LFT's. Get Labs (CBC, CMP, PT/PTT, Type and cross, Lipase, Lactate, RUQ US, possible CT A/P)

3. Diagnosis: Needs ERCP or MRCP.

4. Management: Stat Consult with GI. Give IV Fluids, IV antibiotics. Needs ERCP for Management

4. Cholangitis:

1. Pathology: Infection due to an Obstructed Bile Duct

2. Signs/Symptoms: Fever, RUQ pain, Jaundice ("Charcot's Triad"). When Cholangitis gets even more severe, it turns into "Reynold's pentad" which has the additional features of Altered mental status and Shock/hypotension. Send Labs (CBC, CMP, PT/PTT, Type and cross, Lipase, Lactate, Cultures, Cardiac Enzymes & EKG (if applicable), RUQ US, Possible CT A/P). Increased LFT's, Increased Alkaline Phosphatase, Increased Leukocytes

3. Diagnosis/Management: Needs Stat Surgery/ERCP (Stat Consult Surgery and GI). NPO, IV fluids, IV antibiotics

PANCREAS

1. Pancreatitis:

1. Pathology: Inflammatory reaction of the Pancreas. Two most common causes are Alcohol and Gallstones

2. Signs/Symptoms: Often the Patient has Abdominal Pain (Epigastric) with Radiation to the Back. May also have Nausea, Vomiting

3. Diagnosis: Lipase is Elevated. CT scan Abdomen/Pelvis specifically to ensure No severe complications of pancreatitis and rule out other serious etiologies

4. Management of Mild Pancreatitis is IVF's, NPO, Admission.

5. For those with Gallstones, CBD stones or Cholangitis, Needs ERCP by GI (Stat consult).

6. Necrotizing Pancreatitis: Needs Surgery, IV Antibiotics, Drainage

7. Additional Information: Antibiotics are Not advocated unless there is an Abscess or an Infection or an underlying manifestation of a condition that needs Antibiotics is present. Complications include Pseudocyst, Hemorrhage, Necrosis, Renal Failure, ARDs, Electrolyte abnormalities, GI bleeding

PERITONEUM

1. **Spontaneous Bacterial Peritonitis:**

   1. Pathology: Translocation of Bacteria from the Gut to the Peritoneum, causing Infection in the Peritoneum. Occurs in those with Portal Hypertension (ie. Cirrhosis patients)

   2. Signs/Symptoms: Abdominal Pain, Fever, Ascites, Nausea, Vomiting

   3. Diagnosis: Paracentesis with > 250 Neutrophils in the Peritoneal Fluid

   4. Management: Admit and IV Antibiotics (ie. Cefotaxime)

STOMACH/DUODENUM

1. Peptic Ulcer Disease

a) Pathology: Ulcer in the Stomach or Duodenum. Etiologies: H pylori, NSAID's, Gastrinomas (ie ZES). Types: Gastric, Duodenal

b) Signs/Symptoms: Abdominal pain, Nausea, Vomiting, GI bleed are all possible

c) Diagnosis: Endoscopy is often used in patients with concern for Ulcers, in order to rule out more serious etiologies and find other diagnoses

d) Note that if it's a Perforated Ulcer, it needs a Stat Surgical Consult to go to the OR for Repair (NPO, IVF's, IV antibiotics, Stat Surgery) immediately

e) Management Depends on the Underlying Cause:
   Uncomplicated H. pylori Management (one example of a regimen):
   Metronidazole or Amoxicillin + (PPI) Omeprazole + Clarithromycin

f) Complications: Perforation, Upper GI Bleed

   1) Perforation: Abdominal Pain. Peritoneal Signs on Physical Exam. NPO, Needs IVFs, O2, Monitor, IV Antibiotics, Pain Medications, Antiemetics, Chest X-ray may show Free Air Under the Diaphragm. Stat Surgical consult and Admit to OR. Abdominal pain (severe), Nausea, Vomiting on exam, often Guarding, Rigidity, Rebound Tenderness

   2) Upper GI Bleed: Hematemesis, Melena. Needs IVF's, PRBC's, PPI (ie.

Protonix), Stat GI consult, Endoscopy for Management

2. Pyloric Stenosis:

a) Pathology: Narrowing of the opening between where the stomach and intestine meet, due to a Hypertrophied Pylorus. Mostly occurs in Newborns.

b) Signs/Symptoms: Projectile Vomiting, Lethargy, Decreased appetite, Dehydration

c) Diagnosis: Ultrasound. Labs may show abnormalities (Dehydration or Abnormal Electrolytes), Clinical

d) Management: Stat Surgery Consult. IVF's, Electrolyte correction, Surgery consult for Pylorotomy

3. Foreign Body (Stomach): Most Foreign Bodies that reach the Stomach will pass. Endoscopic Intervention is needed if they are sharp/long/large in size or symptomatic or not progressing along. If asymptomatic and don't have any of the above characteristics, serial X-rays can be taken to ensure that the Foreign Body is progressing along to pass.

4. Gastritis:

5. Pathology: Inflammation of Stomach Lining

6. Signs/Symptoms: Epigastric Pain, Anorexia, Possible Nausea and Vomiting

7. Diagnosis: Endoscopy

8. Treatment: Dependent on the Etiology. Antacids

9. Please note: Generally don't like to come to this diagnosis initially, without first ruling out more serious etiologies, like a Myocardial Infarction. Beware: The symptoms of an MI can also improve with the use of Antacids so be careful not to misdiagnose!

SMALL BOWEL

1. Mesenteric Ischemia:

a) Pathology: Blood Flow to the Intestines are Blocked due to one of the following: An Arterial Embolus (ie. SMA Embolus), Arterial Thrombus (ie. SMA Thrombosis), Low Flow states (ie. Congestive Heart Failure) or a Venous Thrombosis/ Hypercoagulable state (ie. DVT, PE, etc)

b) More Prevalent in Cardiac Patients (Atrial Fibrillation because prone to Emboli), MI patients

c) Signs/Symptoms: Abdominal pain ("Pain out of proportion to physical exam"), Nausea, Vomiting, Possible Bloody Stool

d) Diagnosis: Often Lactate is elevated. CT Abdomen/Pelvis. Angiography

e) Management: Need a Stat Surgery Consult. IVF's, IV antibiotics. Surgery consult, (for ie. Embolectomy, Thrombolysis, etc.)

2. Obstruction (Small Bowel Obstruction "SBO"):

a) Pathology: Blockage of the Small Intestine. Often secondary to Adhesions from Prior Surgeries and Hernias

b) Signs/Symptoms: Abdominal pain, Nausea, Vomiting, Constipation

c) Diagnosis: Abdomen Xray Flat and Erect, CT Abdomen/Pelvis

d) Management: NPO, NG tube, IVF's, Stat Surgery consultation and Admission for Possible Operative Intervention (Complete Obstruction)

3. Paralytic Ileus:

a) Pathology: Functional Disturbance in Physiological Process.

b) Signs/Symptoms: Nausea, Vomiting, Abdominal Pain

c) Diagnosis: CT Abdomen/Pelvis

d) Management: NG tube, IVF's and Treat Underlying Etiology

4. Aortoenteric Fistula:

a) Pathology: Occurs when there is a communication between the Aorta or the region of an Aortic Graft with a portion of the Intestines

b) Signs/Symptoms: Can Present as GI bleed (ie Hematemesis, Hematochezia, etc). Can present with Abdominal pain

c) Diagnosis: CT Abdomen/Pelvis with Contrast, if stable

d) Management: An unstable patient needs STAT surgery for Laparotomy for repair. A Stable patient can have CT scan Abdomen/Pelvis with Contrast. STAT Surgery Consult for repair. If there is any evidence of infection, give Antibiotics as well

5. Crohn's Disease:

a) Pathology: Inflammatory bowel disease

b) Signs/Symptoms: Abdominal Pain, Weight loss, Diarrhea

c) Diagnosis: Colonoscopy. In the ER, do a CT Abdomen/Pelvis.

d) Treatment: Corticosteroids, Antibiotics (for Infection), Immunomodulators. Get a GI Consult. Admit.

e) Complications of Crohn's: SBO, Abscess, Fistula, Cancer

6. Meckel's diverticulum:

a) Pathology: From the embryo, the Vitelline duct remains. Often manifests as Gastric Tissue that is out of place, that causes GI bleeding. Usually by age 2 years old but can occur at any age

b) Signs/Symptoms: GI Bleeding, May or may not cause pain, May also manifest with Obstruction

c) Diagnosis: Meckel's Scan

d) Management: IVF's and Stat Surgery Consult for Surgical Repair

e) Complications of Meckel's include Bowel Obstruction, Hemorrhage, Perforation.

LARGE INTESTINE

1. **Ulcerative Colitis:**

    1. Pathology: Inflammatory Bowel Disease that involves the Colon, Rectum

    2. Signs/Symptoms: Bloody Diarrhea, Abdominal pain

    3. Diagnosis: Colonoscopy. Do CT Abdomen/Pelvis to look for Complications.

    4. Management: GI Consult. Steroids. Sulfasalazine, Corticosteroids, Immunomodulators. Admit.

    5. Additional information: These patients risk of Colon Cancer is increased

    6. Complications: **Toxic Megacolon,** which presents with: Abdominal Pain, Toxic appearing patient, Possible GI Bleed. Do CT Abdomen/Pelvis. Needs Stat Surgery Consult, NPO, IV Antibiotics, NG Tube

2. **Appendicitis:**

    1. Pathology: Occurs secondary to an obstructed Appendix (ie. due to a fecalith)

    2. Signs/Symptoms: Periumbilical pain initially that localizes to the RLQ, Nausea, Vomiting, Anorexia, Fever, Abdominal Pain, Possible Diarrhea

    3. Diagnosis: CT Abdomen/Pelvis (in children consider US RLQ to avoid radiation, if available at institution). Note: Physical exam may show Psoas Sign, Obdurator Sign, Rovsing Sign. Tenderness over McBurney's Point

    4. Management: IVF's, NPO, IV Antibiotics, Stat Surgery consult and Appendectomy in OR

3. **Necrotizing enterocolitis (NEC):**

    1. Pathology: Infection and necrosis of intestinal wall. Often in premature infants

    2. Signs/Symptoms: Bloody diarrhea, Abdominal pain, Vomiting

    3. Diagnosis: Clinical, X-ray

    4. Management: NPO, IV Fluids, IV Antibiotics, Needs Stat Surgery Consult

4. **Radiation colitis:** Occurs Secondary to Radiation Treatment of Abdomen and Pelvis. Patient may have Bloody Diarrhea, Abdominal Pain

5. **Hirschsprung's disease:** Newborn doesn't pass first stool. Needs Surgery Consult for Operative Repair

6. **Large Bowel Obstruction:**

   1. Pathology: Obstruction of Large Bowel

   2. Signs/Symptoms: Abdominal pain and Vomiting. Possible Constipation

   3. Diagnosis is X-ray or CT Abdomen/Pelvis

   4. Management: NPO, IVF's, Antibiotics (if infection or complication of LBO), Stat Surgery Consult needed for Operative intervention

7. **Diverticulitis:**

   1. Pathology: Inflammation of the Diverticula in the Colon

   2. Signs/Symptoms: LLQ pain, N/V, Diarrhea

   3. Diagnosis: CT Abdomen/Pelvis

   4. Management: IVF's, IV Antibiotics (Ciprofloxacin and Flagyl). If a complication exists (Perforation or Abscess), Consult Surgery Stat and Admit.

8. **Intussusception:**

   1. Pathology: Telescoping of the Intestines into itself, usually in a child but can also be seen in adults

   2. Signs/Symptoms: Child often draws up legs while crying in pain, Abdominal pain, Nausea, Vomiting, Possible Blood in Stools, Weakness

   3. Diagnosis: Ultrasound or Contrast Enema (Air Enema) (In Adults: CT scan Abdomen/Pelvis)

   4. Management: Stat Surgery Consult. IR Consult. Air Enema. If Failure of Air Enema, Next Step is Surgical Intervention

5. Note: When is a Barium Enema **Contraindicated**? Perforated Viscous

9. **Volvulus:**

　　1. Pathology: Large Intestine Blockage Secondary to Twisting

　　2. Signs/Symptoms: Abdominal Pain, Nausea, Vomiting

　　3. Diagnosis: X-ray Abdomen or CT Abdomen/Pelvis

　　4. Management: Needs Surgery and GI consult. Diagnosis and Treatment: Sigmoidoscopy, Rectal Tube, Surgical Repair

RECTUM AND ANUS

1. **Perianal Abscess:**

　　1. Pathology: Abscess in the Perianal region

　　2. Signs/Symptoms: Rectal pain. Fluctuant abscess that is present alongside the anus

　　3. Diagnosis: Clinical

　　4. Management: Can be managed in the ER with Incision and Drainage, Antibiotics and Surgery follow up. Admit if the patient is Elderly, Immunocompromised, Toxic appearing, Abnormal Lab Results or Abnormal Vital Signs.

2. **Perirectal abscess:** Ischiorectal, Supralevator, Intersphincteric

　　1. Pathology: Abscess that is Deeper in the Rectal region

　　2. Signs/Symptoms: Rectal pain

　　3. Diagnosis: Clinical, CT Abdomen/Pelvis

　　4. Management: Surgery Consult for OR drainage and Antibiotics

3. **Pilonidal Abscess:**

   1. Pathology: Abscess over Lower Sacral Region

   2. Signs/Symptoms: Rectal Pain, Drainage, Erythema, Pus

   3. Diagnosis: Clinical

   4. Management: Antibiotics, I&D in ER with Surgeon follow up as an outpatient for Excision of it Surgically.

4. **Proctitis:**

   1. Pathology: Inflammation of the Rectum that can be due to Radiation or Injury or Infection or Pathological Disease

   2. Drainage, Pain in the Rectum, Possible Rectal Bleeding

   3. Diagnosis: Clinical, Physical Exam, Anoscopy, Blood tests/Cultures, Sigmoidoscopy, Colonoscopy

   4. Management: Needs Sitz bath, Supportive treatment, Antibiotics or Antivirals if Infection is the source. Treat the Underlying Etiology.

5. **Anal Fissure:**

   1. Pathology: Tear in the skin of the anus

   2. Signs/Symptoms: Rectal bleeding. Very painful rectum while passing stool. Possible minimal blood from rectum

   3. Diagnosis: Clinical

   4. Management: Stool softeners. Sitz baths. Topical nitroglycerin. Surgery follow up

6. **Anal Fistula:**

   1. Pathology: Skin and Anus are Connected

   2. Signs/Symptoms: Purulent Drainage, Pain, Swollen

   3. Diagnosis: Anoscopy or Ultrasound

4. Management: Surgeon Referral, Sitz Bath, may consider Antibiotics

7. Foreign Body:

1. Pathology: Foreign body inserted into rectum

2. Signs/Symptoms: Rectal pain, bleeding, abdominal pain, obstruction

3. Diagnosis: X-ray (to see the details of the foreign body/bodies but also to ensure no disastrous complications like perforation have occurred) pre and post procedure. Need an Xray for all Patients with Rectal Foreign Bodies.

4. Management: May attempt removal if safe to do so and no complications from the foreign body. If there are symptoms or the patient has a complication (ie. perforation, must get a Surgery consultation Stat. Surgical Removal is also needed if the item is pointy/sharp/multiple objects/abnormal shape/Any Complications, etc.

5. Stat Surgical Consult

6. Even if able to remove the Foreign Body in the ER, you must Admit the Patient as they will need to be under Observation and Under the Care of the Surgeon for further testing

8. Hemorrhoids:

1. Pathology: Veins in the rectum/anus are swollen. Types: Internal (painless) vs External (painful)

2. Signs/Symptoms: Bloody stool, Possible Pain (External)

3. Diagnosis: Clinical, Anoscopy

4. Management: Sitz bath, Stool Softener, Surgeon follow up (Surgery consult Stat if necrosis, thrombosed hemorrhoid)

9. Rectal Prolapse:

1. Pathology: Rectum protrudes outward

2. Signs/Symptoms: Pain or No Pain

3. Diagnosis: Clinical

4. Management: If No evidence of ischemia, it must be reduced. Surgeon consultation if unable to reduce or if there is any concern for Ischemia

GI BLEEDING

UPPER GI BLEED

1. Melena, Hematemesis
2. Etiologies: PUD, Esophageal Varices, etc.
3. Management: Airway Management, Breathing, Circulation, IV X 2, O2, Monitor
4. Send all Labs (CBC, CMP, PT/PTT, Type and Cross, etc.), EKG
5. Needs Endoscopy! Consult GI Stat and Surgery Consult Stat
6. Esophageal Varices needs Stat GI Consult for Stat Endoscopy. Give Octreotide and Give IV Antibiotics
7. In UGIB also give PPI (Protonix), as it could be secondary to PUD

LOWER GI BLEED

1. Hematochezia
2. Management: Airway Management, Breathing, Circulation, IV X 2, O2, Monitor
3. Send all Labs (CBC, CMP, PT/PTT, Type and Cross, etc.), EKG
4. Consult GI Stat and Surgery Consult Stat

PERFORATED VISCOUS

1. An Abdominal Organ can Rupture (Stomach, Duodenum, Small Bowel, Large Bowel, etc).

2. This is a Life threatening Emergency.

3. Diagnosis may be visualizable on an Upright CXR that may show Free Air Under the Diaphragm. Diagnosis may even be noted on Physical Exam (May Present with Rebound Tenderness, Guarding (Peritoneal Signs)).

4. Needs a Stat Surgical Consult. The Patient needs to be NPO. Must give the patient IV Fluids, IV Antibiotics and the Patient needs Stat Surgical Intervention

CARDIOPULMONARY ARREST

1. Pulseless Electrical Activity (PEA): IV, O2, Cardiac Monitor. At this time the General Guidelines to PEA Management consist of the following: Check the Rhythm (in PEA there is a Rhythm on the Monitor but No pulse and it is Not Vfib or Vtach). Start CPR (2 minutes). Pulse Check (In PEA there is No pulse). Note that if the Rhythm is demonstrative of a normal rhythm without a pulse...this is PEA! Resume CPR. Give epinephrine q 3 to 5 minutes, but the **Main Management is to find the Reversible cause and Treat it.** The list of reversible causes include: **H**ypoxia, **H**ypovolemia, **H**ypoglycemia, **H**ypothermia, **H**yperkalemia, **H**ypokalemia, **A**cidosis, **T**ension Pneumothorax, **T**hrombosis (Pulmonary Embolism, Myocardial Infarction), Cardiac **T**amponade, **T**oxins (TCA's, etc). A Mnemonic for the Reversible Causes is **HAT.** If Cardiac Tamponade was the Reversible cause, a Pericardiocentesis would need to be done. If the Reversible cause is a Tension Pneumothorax, a Needle Decompression and then a Chest Tube would need to be done and so on so forth. **Mnemonic (for Reversible Causes): HAT**

2. SUID (Sudden Unexpected Infant Death): Those who are under a year old, who suddenly die unexpectedly. How to help prevent this: Sleep on the back (Avoid sleeping supine. Instead, sleep in the prone position). Avoid keeping any other objects in the crib that can prevent the infant from breathing. Avoid sleeping on soft bedding. Avoid excessively warm clothes or temperatures for the infant. Educate the parents of infants about SUID so that they can take all the necessary steps to prevent this from occurring.

ARTERIAL CIRCULATION DISORDERS

1. **AAA (Abdominal Aortic Aneurysm):** Case Scenario: An Elderly Man with a history of HTN, DM, CAD presents with Back pain or Abdominal Pain or Syncope or Possible Hematuria or Numbness/Weakness. An Ultrasound will show an Enlarged Aorta but a CT scan of the Abdomen/Pelvis with IV Contrast will show if the Aorta is Ruptured. Do a CT Abdomen/Pelvis, if Stable. If Unstable and Suspect Ruptured AAA or the Diagnosis of a Ruptured AAA is Confirmed with CT in a Stable patient, then the Patient Needs a Stat Surgery Consult and must go to the OR immediately for Operative Repair! Give IVF's, PRBC's as these patients are often times Hypotensive due to the Rupture. Note: On Physical exam, you may find a Pulsatile Abdominal Mass. You might find a diminished or absent Femoral Pulse. However, all of these do not always have to be present. So when you suspect it, manage it accordingly!

2. **Aortic Dissection:** Pathophysiology: Tear in the Wall of the Aorta leading to a False Lumen in which blood "dissects". Risk Factors = Men, Smokers, HTN, Pregnant women, Trauma. Symptoms = Chest pain, Back pain, Often Sudden Onset and Severe ("Tearing"), Radiates. Often Hypertensive. Syncope. Can have CVA Symptoms (Weakness, Slurred Speech). Can present as a Myocardial Infarction (STEMI), CVA (Stroke), Mesenteric Ischemia. May present as CHF, Heart Block, Aortic Regurgitation. May have Hoarseness, Horner's Syndrome. Patient is usually Hypertensive but can become Hypotensive. May have a Blood Pressure Discrepancy between the two arms. May have Pulse Deficits. Might hear an Aortic Regurgitation Murmur on exam. There may be Neurological Deficits present. Reminder: Reassess the Patient Often. Diagnosis: Chest X-ray may show a Widened Mediastinum and a CTA Chest/Abdomen (If Patient is Stable) will show Aortic Dissection. What to order: CBC, CMP, PT/PTT, T&C, Lactate, D-Dimer, Urinalysis, Cardiac Enzymes, EKG, CXR, CT Chest/Abdomen (if Stable) and TEE (if Unstable). Provide Pain Medications (ie morphine if not allergic). If Hypertensive, give a Beta Blocker (ie. Esmolol or Labetalol) first and then a vasodilator (ie. Nitroprusside). Give the Beta blocker first to Avoid Reflex Tachycardia from worsening the Dissection. Consult Vascular Surgery Stat. Discuss with Vascular Surgeon for OR and then ICU.

Reminder! Always look out for Dissection in a STEMI patient! An Aortic Dissection can cause and present as a STEMI. In these (dissection) patients **Never** administer thrombolytics nor anticoagulants nor plavix nor aspirin. They are all **Contraindicated**! Always use your better judgment and keep your differential for the most detrimental diagnoses in mind!

3. **Arterial Thromboembolism:** It can manifest in different organ systems and results from an Embolus, a Thrombus, etc. (ie. GI tract: Mesenteric Ischemia, Brain: CVA, Extremity: Acute Limb Ischemia, etc.)

3a. **Acute Limb Ischemia:** It is either due to a Thrombus or an Embolus. Causes include Atrial fibrillation, Heart thrombus after an MI etc. Can present with Painful foot, Cold Foot, Paresthesias, Pale foot, Pulseless foot, or Paralysis. An Embolus (ie. from Atrial fibrillation) can cause a Sudden Onset Ischemic Limb. This is very concerning and is an Emergency. If you don't feel a pulse, Use a Doppler Ultrasound to look for a pulse. An ABI calculation (Ankle Brachial Index) often is <0.5 is very concerning. Management: Heparin (unless contraindicated) and Immediate Vascular Surgery Consultation and Interventional Radiology for an Embolectomy, etc.

VENOUS CIRCULATION DISORDERS

1. **Venous Thromboembolism:**

    1. **DVT (Deep vein thrombosis):** Blood Clot in the Deep Veins of Lower Extremity (or Upper Extremity)

    2. **PE (Pulmonary embolism):** Blood Clot in the Lung Vasculature

    3. **Risk factors:** Immobilization (ie Recent Surgery, Long Plane Ride or Car Ride/ Travel), History of DVT or PE, OCP use, Malignancy, Family History of Blood Disorders/Thrombophilias, Smoking, CHF, CVA, Pregnancy, Elderly, Obesity, Recent Trauma

    4. Note: D-Dimer should only be used to try to rule out a chance of PE in patients who are at **LOW** risk for PE. It cannot be used on moderate or high risk patients.

    5. See Chart Below for Symptoms, Diagnosis, Management

DVT	PE
Pain, Swelling, Possible Warmth/Redness. Tenderness possible	Chest pain, Dyspnea
	Possible Syncope/Anxiety, Tachycardia, Tachypnea
Dx: Ultrasound Lower Extremity with Doppler	Dx: CTA chest with contrast to r/o PE or V/Q scan if CTA contraindicated (ie. Renal Failure)
Tx: Anticoagulation	Tx: Anticoagulation

DISTURBANCES OF CARDIAC RHYTHM

1. **Bradycardia**

a. **Sinus Bradycardia:** Slow Hear Rate. Bradycardia Needs Treatment if Symptomatic (see Most Current ACLS Guidelines for Bradycardia). Bradycardia can be caused by Medications (ie. Beta blockers), MI, Hypothyroidism, Hypothermia, etc. May be normal in Athletes.

b. **Symptomatic Bradycardia:** (ie. Chest Pain, Hypotension, CHF, AMS). Per ACLS guidelines, you could start with atropine and if this does not work you could do Transcutaneous Pacing (or give Dopamine or Epinephrine in lieu of this), while awaiting to do Transvenous Pacing, if needed, depending on the scenario.

2.   **Tachyarrhythmia**

a) **SVT (Stable)** —> Valsalva maneuver. If it doesn't work, try Adenosine 6 mg followed by a NS flush. If it doesn't work, try Adenosine 12 mg followed by a NS flush. If it doesn't work, try another Adenosine 12 mg followed by a NS flush. If these measures still don't work, consider other agents like Calcium Channel Blockers, Beta Blockers. **SVT (Unstable)** —> Synchronized Cardioversion

b) **Stable Monomorphic Ventricular Tachycardia** —> See Oral Boards Section
Stable: Give Amiodarone
Unstable:
If Monomorphic Ventricular Tachycardia and the patient has a Pulse, the management is Synchronized Cardioversion
If Pulseless Ventricular Tachycardia, Needs Defibrillation (Follow ACLS guidelines)

c) **Ventricular Fibrillation**— > Defibrillate, Follow ACLS guidelines (CPR, Defibrillation, Epinephrine, etc.)

d) **Pulseless Ventricular Tachycardia** — > Defibrillate, Follow ACLS guidelines (CPR, Defibrillation, Epinephrine, etc.)

e) **Torsades (Polymorphic Ventricular Tachycardia)** —>
Magnesium, Defibrillation, Avoid Precipitants

f) **Atrial Fibrillation, Atrial Flutter** —>
Atrial Fibrillation is "Irregularly Irregular" in which P waves are Not seen
Atrial Flutter is a Regular Rhythm with a Narrow QRS. You see "Sawtooth waves" on EKG
Both have the same General Management Principle
Stable: Needs Rate Control with a Calcium Channel Blocker or Beta Blocker
Unstable: Synchronized Cardioversion

g) **WPW: Wolff Parkinson White Syndrome:** There is an Accessory pathway involved. EKG manifests with a Delta wave ("Slurred upstroke" of the QRS) with a Short PR interval. If the Patient is Stable, Management is Procainamide. If the patient is Unstable, Cardioversion is needed.

h) **Brugada Syndrome:** See Oral Boards Section

i) **Prolonged QT Syndrome:** See Oral Boards Section

3. Conduction disorders

a) AV Blocks:

1. **First Degree AV block:** PR interval is Prolonged

2a. **Second Degree AV block type I (Mobitz I = Wenckebach):** PR interval Progressively Prolongs in length, each time before the Dropped QRS

2b. **Second Degree AV block type II (Mobitz II):** PR intervals are Fixed in length, each time before the Dropped QRS

3. **Third Degree AV block:** AV dissociation. Complete Heart Block. Atria and Ventricles are Independent of one another. No Relation between the P's and QRS's

c) Management:

1. **First Degree Block:** Mostly Asymptomatic. If Asymptomatic, No management needed in these scenarios

2. **Second Degree Type I (Mobitz I, Wenckebach),** with Symptoms, Atropine can be given initially. If unstable, consider Pacing

3. **Second Degree Type II (Mobitz II):** Pacemaker (because this can degenerate into a third degree heart block)

4. **Third Degree Heart Block:** Pacemaker

5. AV blocks can be due to an MI but can also be due to Medications (ie Beta Blockers), Hypothermia and Electrolyte Disturbances. Various pathologies can lead to AV Blocks (ie. Lyme disease, etc.)

4. Bundle Branch Blocks:

a) **Left Bundle Branch Block:** Wide QRS. Deep S wave in V1. Broad R wave in I, avL, V5, V6

b) **Right Bundle Branch Block:** Wide QRS. "RSR" Pattern in V1.

DISEASES OF THE MYOCARDIUM

1. Hypertrophic Cardiomyopathy: (HOCM): Sudden Death in young patients who often times have a Family history of Sudden Cardiac Death. May have Dyspnea on Exertion, Syncope, Chest Pain. The Physical Exam may show a Systolic Ejection Murmur. Note: In your Differential Diagnostic search in Young People with Syncope, always ask about any Sudden Early Cardiac Related Death in the Family History! Always think of this Diagnosis! Echocardiogram is the Diagnostic study as it shows a Very Thick Septum. Management: Cardiology Consult, Medications (ie. Beta Blockers), AICD, Operative Repair. Admit.

2. Congestive Heart Failure (CHF): Fluid Overload. Edema (Peripheral), PND (Paroxysmal Nocturnal Dyspnea), Orthopnea, DOE (Dyspnea on Exertion). Etiologies: MI, PE, Valve Dysfunction, Infection, Cardiac issues, etc. Diagnosis: Pro-BNP, CXR (May show Pulmonary Edema, Cephalization, Cardiomegaly, etc. or may initially look normal, when it is too early on), and Echocardiogram. Management is Oxygen, Nitrates (Nitroglycerin), Lasix. If Trouble Breathing despite Oxygen, Bipap can be started, as long as the patient is alert. If deteriorating even on Bipap and decompensating, consider Intubation. Admit.

3. Ischemic Heart Disease: Risk Factors are Smoking, Family History of Early MI; DM, HTN, HLD, Elderly, Men. Note that the Classic Presentation of Pressure like Chest Pain with Radiation to the Bilateral Shoulders or the Left Arm is only seen in some patients but the History does not have to be typical in order to be an MI. In any patient with Moderate to High Risk, get Serial EKG's, Serial Troponins/Cardiac Enzymes and Admit to Observation at the least or Disposition accordingly (ie. STEMI goes for PCI). Note that a good number of patients (Especially Women, Older patients and Diabetics) with MI can have Atypical symptoms such as Dyspnea, Weakness, Nontypical Chest Pain, Epigastric Pain, Diaphoresis, etc. so always keep ACS/MI on your Differential! EKG, Labs (Cardiac Enzymes, etc) and Cardiology Consult. Admit.

a) **Unstable Angina:** Ischemia that is often Worsened at Rest and Worsens in general. EKG does not have obvious ischemic changes and there are Negative cardiac enzymes. O2, ASA, NTG, Anticoagulation (if no contraindications). Cardiology Consult. Admit.

b) **NSTEMI:** EKG does **Not** have ST Elevation on EKG, but may have T wave Inversions or Nonspecific Changes or be Normal. Troponin is Positive. Cardiology Consult. Admit.

c) Management of **STEMI:** Oxygen, Aspirin, Nitroglycerin (Contraindicated in Inferior wall MI), Morphine (Contraindicated in Inferior wall MI), Anticoagulation (Heparin or

Lovenox), GIIb/IIIa inhibitor and Stat Cath lab activation (PCI)

d) **STEMI:** ST Elevation MI on EKG needs PCI preferably (PCI is best). In a facility without easy access to a PCI facility, can consider thrombolytics if there are no contraindications, but do keep in mind that PCI is the Best!

e) **Myocardial infarction:** Coronary Artery Occlusion that leads to myocardial cell death in that region of the heart. Early MI changes on EKG: Hyperacute T waves. This can then become an ST Elevation. Afterwards, T wave inversions and Q waves. In patients with Chest Pain (or any concerning symptoms), always get an EKG and repeat because you want to be able to catch Evolving Changes of an MI before it's too late!

f) **Inferior wall MI:** ST Elevations in at least two contiguous leads in II, III, aVF with Reciprocal ST Depressions in I, aVL. Do a Right sided EKG leads V3R, V4R (ST Elevations in these) to see if there is a Right Ventricular Infarction. In the event of a Right Ventricular Infarction, Give IV Fluids since the Patient is Preload Dependent and give Aspirin. Activate the Cath lab stat. Do **NOT** give anything that can Reduce Preload/Reduce BP or HR (**Contraindicated:** Nitroglycerin, Diuretics and Morphine are all Contraindicated in patients with Right Ventricular Infarction! Also Avoid Beta Blockers in these patients).

g) **Posterior wall MI:** ST Depressions in V1, V2, V3. May also show Tall R waves in these leads. Often times you may only see it in two of these leads. Do EKG with Posterior leads (V7, V8, V9) to see if there are ST elevations in these. Keep in mind that these patients at times present concomitantly with Inferior wall MI's.

h) **Anterior wall MI:** ST Elevations in at least two contiguous leads in V1-V4 with ST Depressions in II, III, aVF

i)   **Lateral wall MI:** I, aVL, V5, V6 has ST elevations and there are ST depressions in II, III, aVF

j) With the **<u>Exception</u>** of Inferior wall MI/Right Ventricular Involvement, in which Nitroglycerin and Morphine are both Contraindicated, the Management of the other forms of STEMI (ie anterior, lateral, septal) is Oxygen, Aspirin, Nitroglycerin, Morphine, Anticoagulation (Heparin or Lovenox), GIIb/IIIa inhibitor, PCI

k) What are the **Complications** of an MI? Cardiogenic Shock, Arrhythmias, Pericarditis, Cardiac Tamponade, CHF, Ventricular Aneurysm, Myocardial Rupture (ie. LV Rupture), Mitral Regurgitation

l) **Ventricular Aneurysm:** On EKG shows ST elevation. Occurs after an MI. Diagnosis is Echocardiogram

m) **Rupture of LV:** Chest pain. Diagnosis is Echocardiogram. Management is Stat Surgical Intervention. Has a High Mortality Rate.

4. **Myocarditis:** Inflammation of the Myocardium. Elevated Cardiac Enzymes (Troponin). Can manifest with Chest pain, Fever, Recent URI, Dyspnea, Palpitations. Management is Supportive and to treat the Symptoms/Presentation (ie. if it manifests as CHF, it needs treatment for this). Admit all Patients for Monitoring, Repeat Labwork, Further Testing (Echo) to ensure that No Cardiac Complications Occur.

DISEASES OF THE PERICARDIUM

1. **Pericardial Tamponade:** Cardiac Tamponade. Fluid/Blood around the Heart. Symptoms/Signs that comprise the Classic Beck's Triad: JVD, Muffled Heart Sounds/Distant Heart Sounds and Hypotension. May see Electrical Alterans (Low Voltage) on EKG. Pulses Paradoxes (Drop in SBP by 10 with Inspiration). May see Cardiomegaly or a Water Bottle sign on CXR. Needs a Echocardiogram. Management is an IV Fluid Bolus, Pericardiocentesis. Cardiothoracic Surgery Consult for a Pericardial Window. ICU Admission.

2. **Pericarditis:** Inflammation of the Pericardium (Can be secondary to an Infection from a Virus/Bacteria or Radiation or Uremia or a Comorbidity (ie. Lupus) or a Malignancy or a Medication). Can also Occur after an MI. Possible prior URI, Fever, Chest pain (often sharp) that is worse with laying Supine and better sitting up/forward. May hear a Friction Rub when auscultating the heart. EKG with STE diffusely (not in avR) possible and PR depression (not in avR). May have Flat or Inverted T waves. May have a Normal EKG. Diagnosis is Echocardiogram to make sure that there is no Pericardial Effusion/Cardiac Tamponade. Treatment: NSAID. Antibiotics if infectious etiology. Admit if symptomatic, abnormal vital signs, abnormal labs, comorbidities, on anticoagulation, history of trauma, effusion/tamponade, infection or any other concerning findings. Generally, one should Admit Patients with Pericarditis. Note: Patients with Uremic Pericarditis need Dialysis.

DISEASES OF THE ENDOCARDIUM

1. **Infectious Endocarditis (IE):** Inflammation/Infection of the Endothelium of the Heart/Valves. Presents with a Murmur + Fever. May have Janeway lesions, Roth spots, Osler nodes, Splinter Hemorrhages. May present with a Stroke secondary to Emboli. May present with CHF. May present with Kidney issues (ie. Hematuria). Send Labs, Blood Cultures, Urine, etc. Diagnosis: Positive Blood Cultures,

Echocardiogram. Management: Give IV Antibiotics. Admit. Note: Provide Prophylaxis for those undergoing Procedures that could lead to Endocarditis. Patients at Higher Risk include those with Cardiac Transplants, History of IE, Those Undergoing Certain Procedures, those with a history of any type of Heart Disease, IV Drug Abusers, those with Valve Damage/Replacement, etc.

Note: Patients with Lupus can have a Nonbacterial form of Endocarditis (Libman Sacks Endocarditis)

VALVULAR DISORDERS

1. **Aortic Stenosis:** Systolic Murmur. May present with Syncope, Chest Pain, CHF (DOE, Orthopnea, PND, etc). Can cause death. Diagnosis: Echocardiogram. Admit if Symptomatic. Cardiology Consult. Management is Aortic Valve Replacement. Please Note the Following: Do **Not** give these patients any Medications that can lower their Preload.

2. **Mitral Regurgitation:** Systolic Murmur. May manifest with CHF symptoms: SOB, DOE, Orthopnea, Pulmonary Edema. Needs a Cardiology Consult. Diagnosis: Echocardiogram. Cardiology Consult. Needs Mitral Valve Replacement. Note: If the patient is Unstable, consider an MI being the cause of the MR and needs Cardio, Cath Lab. MR can present after an MI.

3. **Aortic Regurgitation:** Diastolic Murmur. Keep in mind that this murmur an be seen in patients with pathologies like Aortic Dissection and Endocarditis. May present with CHF, Chest Pain, SOB. Diagnosis: Echocardiogram. Cardiology Consult. Needs Stat Surgical Intervention.

4. **Mitral Stenosis:** Diastolic Murmur. May present with Dyspnea, Chest Pain, Hemoptysis, CHF, etc. Diagnosis: Echocardiogram. Cardiology Consult. Admit. Management: Mitral valve replacement if Symptomatic/Severe symptoms is the Definitive Management. Etiology often is Rheumatic Heart Disease. May also find Atrial Fibrillation and Embolization in these patients.

HYPERTENSIVE EMERGENCIES
1. Hypertension along with End Organ Damage
2. It can manifest as Hypertensive Encephalopathy, Eclampsia, Stroke, Myocardial infarction, Aortic Dissection, CHF, Pulmonary Edema, Pheochromocytoma, Acute Renal Failure. These Need Management with the Appropriate Agents and Needs Admission.
3. Aortic Dissection: Beta Blocker first (ie. Esmolol) and then Nitroprusside
4. Pheochromocytoma: Phentolamine
5. Eclampsia: Magnesium must be given. If the patient is still Hypertensive, may add on either Hydralazine or Labetalol

DERMATOLOGIC DISORDERS

MACULOPAPULAR LESIONS

1. **Erythema Multiforme:** Target lesions. Can occur after Medication use (ie Antibiotics, Antiepileptics, Nsaid's, etc.) or Viruses (ie. Herpes) or Malignancies or Autoimmune diseases. Treat the Cause. Discontinue the Medication causing it.

2. **Erythema Nodosum:** Occurs in Sarcoidosis and other conditions. An Erythematous, Painful and Nodular lesion that is usually on Pretibial area of legs. Inflammation. May also present with Joint Aches/Muscle Aches
Treatment is Supportive. Treat the Underlying Disorder.

3. **Henoch-Schönlein Purpura (HSP):** Vasculitis of the Lower Extremities and the Buttocks manifesting as Purpura. Can also manifest with Renal issues, Joint pain and Abdominal pain in addition to the Rash. Usually occurs in Children. May have had a URI prior to the manifestation of the HSP. Management is Supportive if Uncomplicated HSP. However, if there is any indication of Renal issues, GI issues or any concerning symptoms, Admit and Consider Steroids.

4. **Pityriasis Rosea:** A Light Pink/Light Orange Oval Patch on the Skin. "Herald Patch" with "Christmas Tree Distribution" of a Pink Rash over the Trunk and the Extremities. Management: Supportive Care

5. **Urticaria:** Hives, Pruritic Elevated Erythematous lesions, Must Assess Airway to ensure it will not close off due to swelling. Often due to Medications, Foods, Dust/Animal Dander. Note that if a Patient has Anaphylaxis the Management is: Epinephrine, Benadryl, Steroids, Albuterol Nebulizer (to Bronchodilate) and an H2 blocker (ie. Ranitidine) to work in synchrony with the H1 blocker. Observe for at least 6 hours to ensure No rebound. If Anaphylaxis or No improvement, then the patient needs Admission. Reminder - Educate patient to avoid the triggering agent. If Patient has Mild urticaria (Mild allergic reaction), try benadryl, steroids and observe for at least 4 to 6 hours to ensure that there is full resolution, no worsening and no new symptoms.

VESICULAR/BULLOUS LESIONS

1. **Pemphigus Vulgaris** - Blistering disorder. Flaccid Bullae. Positive Nikolsky sign (Skin peels off with touching). The majority of patients will have lesions in their Mouth. The diagnosis is a biopsy of the skin to find an antibody specific to Pemphigus. Treatment: Corticosteroids and other immunosuppressants. Admit.

2. **Bullous Pemphigoid** - Autoimmune. Blister formation. Elderly patients. Often Tense Bullae. **Don't** burst them because it will predispose to infection. Negative Nikolsky sign. Diagnosis is the Biopsy of the Skin. Treatment is Corticosteroids and other immunosuppressants. If severe, Admit.

3. **Stevens-Johnson Syndrome** - Sites like the Eyes (Conjunctivae) and the Mouth are involved. Target lesions are present. Involves at least two mucosal sites (mouth, eyes, genitals, etc). Often due to Medications (ie Antibiotics like Sulfa Medications). Treatment: Stop the medication immediately. IVF's. ICU or Burn unit admission.

4. **Toxic Epidermal Necrolysis** - Occurs in adults. Involves >30% of the Total Body Surface Area. Often due to Medications (ie. Antibiotics, Antiepileptics, NSAIDs) and is the worsening form of SJS. Fever, Lethargy, Painful skin lesions. Redness, Blisters, Desquamation. Positive Nikolsky sign. Mouth is involved in the majority of cases. High Mortality. Treatment: Stop the medication that's causing it, Burn Center Transfer/Burn Unit Admission, IV Fluids, Prevent infection

EXOTOXIN FORMATION

1. **Toxic Shock Syndrome** - Due to Staph Aureus. Exotoxin formation. Rash, Desquamation, Fever, Fatigue, Myalgias, Rash looks like a sunburn, Hypotension. Many organ systems involved (Renal, CNS, GI, Liver, etc). Often secondary to Tampon use/Nasal Packing. Management is the Removal of the Tampon/Nasal Packing. IV Antibiotics. IVF's. Admit to the ICU.

2. **Staphylococcal Scalded Skin Syndrome** - Occurs in Children. Due to an Exotoxin. Fever, Rash, Lethargy, Painful Skin Lesions. Red, Tender skin. Desquamation and Bullae. Positive Nikolsky sign (Skin peels off with touching). Treatment: IVF's, IV Antibiotics and Admit to the ICU.

ULCERATIVE LESIONS

1. **Decubitus Ulcer:** Often occurs in patients who remain stationary (ie nursing home patients who are unfortunately not turned around every 2 hours). Often occurs in regions such as the lower back (ie. sacrum). Different stages exist: I = Erythema, II = Epidermis involvement, III = Dermis and Subcutaneous tissue involvement, IV = Fascia, Bone, Muscle possibly involved. Prevention: Change Patients Position every 2 hours to avoid pressure ulcers from forming. Treatment = Special Dressings, Possible Debridement/Surgical Intervention for Stages III, IV. Specialty Follow Up or Consult depending on the Presentation. Consider Antibiotics.

SKIN INFECTIONS

1. **Abscess:** Erythema, Fluctuance. Tenderness. If Palpable Fluctuance is present, needs I&D. Needs Incision and Drainage and Antibiotics

2. **Cellulitis:** Erythema, Warmth, Tenderness. Needs Antibiotics. Of note: US Venous Doppler Lower Extremity if concern for DVT

3. **Erysipelas:** Erythema often of the Cheeks or Legs. Possible Lethargy and Fever. Management: Antibiotics. Generally, Admit.

4. **Scarlet Fever:** Fever, Sore throat. Often due to Group A Strep. Presents with a "Sandpaper" like rash. May also present with Pastia's lines and a Strawberry Tongue. Treatment is Penicillin.

5. **Impetigo:** Small Vesicles or Yellow crusted lesions often around the mouth in children usually. Treatment is Topical Mupirocin. If complicated, can use PO Antibiotic.

6. **Necrotizing Fasciitis:** A Very Dangerous Infection. Anaerobic organisms often prevalent. "Pain out of Proportion to Exam". Excruciating Pain. Bullae. Fever. Painful. May have Crepitus. Infection travels through the Fascia. Management is Immediate Surgical Consult and Debridement and IV Antibiotics.

7. **Herpes Simplex:** Vesicular Rash. Often either on the Mouth or the Genital area. Treatment is Acyclovir.

8. **Herpes Zoster:** A Painful Vesicular Rash that is along a Single Dermatome (unless immunocompromised, then may be along Multiple Dermatomes). Management is Acyclovir or Valacyclovir.

9. **Scabies:** Due to Mites. Itchy Rash often along the Webspace of the Hands. Treatment is Permethrin cream, Wash all linen in Hot water.

10. **RMSF (Rocky Mountain Spotted Fever):** Tick Bite usually (Patient may not know it), Headache, Fever, Fatigue, Myalgias, Rash (Maculopapular) that starts on the wrists, ankles and then spreads to the trunk, palms, soles. Name is a misnomer as it really occurs more in the Southeast rather than the Rocky's. Treatment is Doxycycline.

11. **Rubella:** Lymphadenopathy (ie Postauricular), Rash. Management: Supportive

12. **Measles:** Rhinorrhea, Conjunctivitis. Rash. Koplik Spots on the Mouth.

Management is Supportive. Also Known as Rubeola.

13. Erythema Infectiosum: "Slapped Cheek": Both cheeks look Red on the Child. Generalized weakness. Management is Supportive. If an adult catches the Parvovirus that causes this, they can get Arthritis.

14. Molluscum Contagiosum: Due to Poxvirus. Umbilicated Papules. Contagious. Often self limiting. May have to treat the underlying precipitant.

DERMATITIS

1. Atopic: Occurs in those with Asthma or Eczema family history. Pruritic Rash. Tx: Avoid inciting factors. Give Moisturizers, Topical Steroids, etc.

2. Contact: Due to Plants, Jewelry, Clothes or New Lotion/Soaps Exposure to Skin. Treatment: Avoid the cause. Wash Current Clothes and Beddings, Benadryl, Oatmeal Bath, Steroids

3. Psoriasis: Presents with Scale like Plaques on the Extensors Regions of the Body. Management is Topical or Systemic Steroids, MTX, Phototherapy

FUNGAL

1. Tinea: Skin infections that can occur on the Head, Body, Feet and may manifest as Circular scale covered demarcations. Treatment is Antifungal Agent

SKIN CANCER

1. **Basal Cell Carcinoma:** Often in Elderly patients who have had sun exposure. Looks like a white nodule. Often on the face/forehead. Needs a Dermatologist for a Biopsy and then Surgical excision and further necessary treatments

2. **Kaposi's Sarcoma:** Often occurs in HIV patients; looks like a purple colored skin rash with plaques or papular in quality located on the body. Must treat patients with HIV with the HAART regimen

3. **Melanoma:** Most deadly skin cancer. A mole that changes in color, size (enlarges), shape (irregular borders), quality are all concerning. Diagnosis is Dermatology for a Biopsy. If early on, resection. If later in stage (ie metastases), chemotherapy and radiation may be needed

4. **Squamous Cell Carcinoma:** Also looks like a nodule. Looks slightly ulcerated. Needs a Dermatologist for a Biopsy. Treatment is often Resection

ENDOCRINE, METABOLIC

ADRENAL DISEASE

1. **Corticoadrenal Insufficiency:** Deficiency of Corticosteroids. Adrenal crisis is a life threatening emergency. Patients may present with Weakness, Hypotension, Abdominal pain, Nausea, Vomiting. Often occurs in those with Chronic Steroid use who are abruptly withdrawn from it. Primary Adrenal Insufficiency: Hyperkalemia, Hyponatremia, Hypoglycemia, Hyperpigmented Skin. Send Cortisol Level. Management is IV fluids, Steroids (Dexamethasone or Hydrocortisone). Treat the Underlying Cause (ie Infection). Treat Underlying Electrolyte Disorders.

2. **Cushing's Syndrome:** Caused by Excess levels of Glucocorticoids. Results in Moon Facies, Obesity, HTN, DM, Hirsutism, Possible Amenorrhea, Possible Psychological Conditions, Osteoporosis, Weakness. Management: Treat the Underlying Cause and try to progressively discontinue the steroids

ELECTROLYTE DISTURBANCES

1. **Hypercalcemia: H**eart block, Short QT, **P**ain in Joints/Bones, Kidney Stones, **W**eakness, **A**MS, **A**bdominal Pain, **R**enal stones, **V**omiting, **A**bdominal pain, **N**ausea; Management is **Fluids   Mnemonic: HOP** onto the **WAR VAN** but bring **FLUIDS**

2. **Hypocalcemia: W**eakness, **D**ysrhythmias, **P**aresthesias, **N**umbness, **T**etany, Hyperreflexia. Management is Calcium   **Mnemonic: WED PANT**

3. **Hypokalemia:** Weakness, Dysrhythmias, Possible Vomiting. Tx is Potassium (Oral is Safer to use, as long as patient is stable and the level is not extremely low). Check Magnesium Level as well because many times the patient is hypomagnesemic as well and if this is the case, must supplement. Correct a Low Magnesium as well in order for the Potassium correction for Hypokalemia to be effective.

4. **Hyperkalemia:** Weakness, Dysrhythmias. EKG: No P wave, Peaked T waves, Wide QRS. Management: **C**alcium gluconate, **I**nsulin, Sodium **B**icarbonate, **A**lbuterol, **D**extrose, **K**ayexalate (and Dialysis in renal failure patients on dialysis, etc).
Admit. **Mnemonic for Hyperkalemia Treatment is: C I (see) a BAD K**

5. **Hyponatremia:** Weakness, AMS, Confusion, Seizure, Headache, N/V. Management: Water Restriction if patient is Hypervolemic. If

Hypovolemic, can give Fluids. If very low Sodium level or the patient has a Seizure, Confusion or Severe Neurological symptoms, Consider Hypertonic Saline (but give it very slowly in order to avoid complications like Cerebral Pontine Myelinosis). Needs ICU admission. Admit.

6. **Hypernatremia:** AMS, Seizure, Weakness, Dehydration, N/V. Needs Slow correction with Fluids (Give Slowly to Avoid Cerebral Edema). Admit

7. **Hypermagnesemia:** Weakness, Nausea, Vomiting, AMS, Loss of DTR's. Respiratory Distress. Dysrhythmia. Management: Hydration. If severe, consider Calcium. Diuretics. In Renal Patients, Hemodialysis. Admit

8. **Hypomagnesemia:** Can cause Dysrhythmias. Increased Reflexes. Can cause a Seizure, Weakness, Tetany, AMS, Dysrhythmia, Tremor. If Mild symptoms or No symptoms: Oral replenishment. If Moderate symptoms: IV Magnesium. If Severe symptoms, need IV Magnesium.

9. **Hypophosphatemia:** AMS, Seizure, Weakness, Respiratory Distress. Cardiac issues. Admit. Repletion. Oral if Moderate, IV if Severe

10. **Hyperphoshatemia:** Numbness, Tetany, Weakness. Manifests like Hypocalcemia because too much Phosphate ends up binding the Calcium. Management is Normal Saline (if renal functioning is normal; if not and patient has Renal Failure, needs hemodialysis), Calcium for Hypocalcemia, and Insulin with Glucose is also needed for Management in this Scenario.

GLUCOSE METABOLISM DISTURBANCES

1. **Type I Diabetes:** Insulin deficiency

2. **Type II Diabetes:** Insulin present but the Receptors are Not sensitive to the Insulin

3. **Hyperglycemia**

a) **Hyperosmolar Hyperglycemic State (HHS):** Possible AMS, Dehydration. Glucose very high, >600, Normal Bicarbonate, Normal pH, No ketosis, Serum osmolality > 315. Management: IVF's (NS) and Insulin. Manage and Treat the Underlying Etiology (Infection, etc).

b) **Diabetic Ketoacidosis (DKA):** Causes of DKA include: MI, Pregnancy, Infection (ie UTI), PE, Hyperthyroidsim, etc). Serum glucose > 250, pH <7.3, Bicarbonate <15 and Ketonemia, Ketonuria. Treatment is IV Fluids (NS), Insulin, Treat the underlying cause (ie Antibiotics for Infection) and the Electrolyte abnormalities.

Note that when the Glucose drops below 250, change the fluids to D5 1/2NS, Check the FSG, CMP and the ABG Hourly (Goal: To close the Anion Gap, etc).

4. **Hypoglycemia:** Causes Weakness, Lethargy, Syncope, Confusion/AMS, Dizziness, Headache, Irritability. Correct with Food, Dextrose. If due to a Moderate or Long Acting insulin or a Sulfonylurea, needs Admission to Prevent Rebound Hypoglycemia from occurring. If due to a Sulfonylurea, give Dextrose, Octreotide and Admit.

NUTRITIONAL DISORDERS

1. **Wernicke-Korsakoff Syndrome:** Often in Alcoholics. It causes Confusion, Ataxia, Ophthalmoplegia, Amnesia and the patient may make up words. Needs Thiamine (Note that one should always give Thiamine before Glucose), Glucose

THYROID DISORDERS

1. **Hyperthyroidism:** The concerning finding with this would be a Thyroid Storm. Palpitations, Exophthalmos, Heat intolerance, Weakness, Tremor, Anxiety, GI issues, Tachycardia, Fever, Arrhythmias, Nausea/Vomiting, Diarrhea, AMS, CHF, Afib (Note: Elderly may only have AMS or Weakness). Primary: TSH (low) and T4 (high) level. Send EKG, Labs, etc.

2. **Thyroid Storm:** Palpitations, AMS, Tachycardia, Febrile, Proptosis, Anxious. Keep ABC's in mind from the get-go for management. Treatment: Airway Management. Management is Beta-blocker (Propranolol) will Block the Peripheral effects of Thyroid Hormone, PTU (Inhibits New Thyroid Hormone Formation) or Methimazole, Iodide One Hour after PTU or Methimazole (Iodide will Inhibit Thyroid Hormone Release) and Corticosteroid (Hydrocortisone or Dexamethasone). ICU Admit for Thyroid Storm.

3. **Apathetic Hyperthyroidism:** Elderly patients with Weakness or AMS who has Hyperthyroidism

3. **Hypothyroidism:** Weakness, Cold Intolerance, Weight Gain, Edema, Constipation, Bradycardia, Hypothermia. Send EKG, Labs, etc. Send Cortisol level. Send TSH, T4. Primary: T4 is low, TSH is high. Send Cortisol level as well in the event of concomitant Adrenal Insufficiency.

4. **Myxedema coma:** AMS, Bradycardia, Hypotensive, Hypothermia, Decreased Reflexes, Edema. Keep ABC's in mind from the get-go for Management (Airway). Treatment is IVF's, Hydrocortisone and Levothyroxine (T4). Treat the underlying cause (ie. If Infection with Antibiotics, etc). Correct Hypothermia, Correct

Electrolytes (ie. Correct Low Glucose with Dextrose), Hydrocortisone (in case Adrenal Insufficiency present as well). ICU Admit. Possible Precipitants: Infection, PE, MI, etc.

METABOLIC ACIDOSIS

1. Mnemonic: **UR DIMPLES**

2. **Causes High Anion Gap Metabolic Acidosis**

3. **Uremia, DKA, Iron, Isoniazid, Metformin, Methanol, Propylene Glycol, Lactic Acidosis, Ethylene Glycol, Ethanol, Salicylates**

PHEOCHROMOCYTOMA

1. Tumor that leads to Catecholamine excess
2. Symptoms include: Anxiety, Flushing, Palpitations, Diaphoresis, Headache
3. Diagnosis: 24 hour urine to test for Catecholamines
4. Management: Phenoxybenzamine (or Phentolamine) which are both Alpha Adrenergic Blockers and thereafter, consider Surgical Management

ENVIRONMENTAL DISORDERS

ANIMAL BITES:

1. **Bees:** Remove Stinger. Benadryl, Tetanus shot, Allergic Reaction Treatments are necessary (ie if Anaphylaxis: Epinephrine, Benadryl, Ranitidine, Albuterol, Steroids. IVF's if Hypotension and if anticipated airway issues (ie edema) then consider intubation). Admit if Moderate to Severe Reaction or any other concerns.

2. **Black Widow Spider:** Neurotoxin. HTN, Tachycardia, Abdominal pain, Severe Myalgias, Nausea, Vomiting. Give Tetanus shot, Pain medications (ie. Morphine), Lorazepam. Antivenin. Admit.

3. **Brown Recluse Spider:** Wound Necrosis. Eschar. Fever. Nausea/Vomiting. Tx is Supportive, Wound Management, Tetanus shot, Pain medications. May Consider Dapsone.

4. For **Animal Bites:** Irrigate the Wound, Get an X-ray, Give a Tetanus shot, Rabies Prophylaxis depending on the animal and region/risk and Start Antibiotics. Always need wound checked.

5. **Cat Bite:** Has the Highest chance of infection. Needs Irrigation, Clean the wound, Tetanus shot, Antibiotics (ie Augmentin)

6. **Human Bite:** Needs Antibiotics (ie. Augmentin). Always ascertain whether patient has a "fight bite" (patient punched the mouth/teeth of another person with his/her fist. Often times the patient's history will not outrightly suggest the true mechanism of injury). For a fight bite the patient needs Irrigation, IV Antibiotics, Hand Surgery/ Orthopedic Consult Stat and Admission. For a Human Bite, otherwise, get an X-ray, Irrigate, give a tetanus shot and one treatment that is often used is Augmentin but if the patient has a penicillin allergy, clindamycin and bactrim may be considered.

7. **Dog Bite:** Give Tetanus shot, Clean the wound, Irrigate, Give Antibiotic as well

8. Any patient with a Cat bite or Human bite, Elderly, Malnourished, HIV, DM (or any Immunocompromised state), Any Bite to the Hand, Joints, Legs, Feet, or Face, Present later than ideal time frame, Artificial valves, Open Fractures, Exposed Tendon/Bone or any other Peripheral Arterial Disease, surely need antibiotics because the Risk of Infection is High

9. **Jellyfish,** Corals are **Nematocysts:** Excruciating Pain, Nausea, Vomiting, Respiratory issues, Cardiac issues (Arrest). Place Vinegar. on the Site. Symptomatic Treatment. Observation to ensure No Systemic involvement ensues.

10. **Stingrays** are **Stingers** that cause Nausea, Vomiting, Respiratory issues, Cardiac issues. Place Hot Water on the lesion and Remove the Foreign Body after an X-ray. Tetanus shot. Antibiotics.

11. **Coral Snake (Elapidae)**- Weakness, Numbness, Severe Neurological Symptoms, Respiratory Paralysis, Double Vision. Poison control. Manage Airway. Needs Antivenin. IVF's. Admit for Monitoring to ensure No Development of Systemic Symptoms.

12. **Rattlesnake (Viper)** - Pain, Bullae, Swollen, Redness over the lesion. May have Systemic changes. May have Coagulopathy. Poison Control. Antivenin. Admit to Observation for Monitoring

DYSBARISM

1. **Types of Barotrauma Mnemonic:**

2. **Mnemonic: PAGE FIRST MD**

3. **P**ulmonary Barotrauma and **A**rterial **G**as **E**mbolism are Barotrauma of Ascent), **F**ace Barotrauma (Face mask squeeze), **I**nner ear ba**R**otrauma, **S**inus baro**T**rauma, **MiD**dle Ear barotrauma

4. **Middle Ear Barotrauma:** Ear Pain, Hearing Loss, Vertigo, Tinnitus, Possible TM Rupture. Tx: Decongestants, Antibiotics

5. **Inner Ear Barotrauma:** Ear Pain, Hearing Loss, Vertigo, Tinnitus. Needs ENT

6. **Sinus Barotrauma:** Facial pain, Headache, Congestion, Sinus pain Epistaxis. Possible Treatment: Decongestants, Antibiotics

7. **Face Barotrauma:** Subconjunctival Hemorrhage

8. **Pulmonary Barotrauma:** Shortness of Breath, Chest Pain, Crepitus (Pneumomediastinum), Pneumothorax (Simple, Tension)

9. **Air Gas Embolism:** Stroke symptoms (Weakness, etc), Possible Myocardial Infarction, AMS, Possible Seizure. This is due to an Air embolus. Occurs with Ascent. Air entry into the Lung vasculature subsequently causing Air Embolus to the Brain (Stroke, Neurological symptoms, Seizure, AMS) or Air Embolus to the Heart (MI). Management: Give 100% Oxygen, Hyperbaric Oxygen Chamber, etc.

10. **Decompression Syndrome:**

a) **Type 1** is The Bends (Joint pain and Tenderness). Arthralgias, Skin Changes

b) **Type 2** Involves Neurological, Pulmonary. Involves: Shortness of Breath, Chest Pain, Back Pain, Cough, Ataxia, Neurological symptoms (Headache, AMS, Seizure, Weakness, etc.), ENT symptoms (Nausea, Vomiting), Eye symptoms (Vision change)

c) Do workup (All Labs, EKG, CXR, CT). Management: Airway, IVF's, 100% O2, Hyperbaric chamber

ELECTRICAL INJURY

1. **Lightning Strike:** Can present with Seizure, AMS, TM rupture, Cardiac Arrest, Dysrhythmias, Loss of consciousness, ICH, Renal failure, Rhabdomyolysis, Trauma. Lichtenberg sign (Ferning pattern) on Skin. IV, O2, Monitor. Physical exam, Labs (CBC, CMP, Cardiac enzymes, CPK, etc.) EKG, CXR, CT, Tetanus shot, Airway. Fluids. Look for Hidden injuries (Trauma evaluation). Reminder: if a patient is in cardiac arrest you should resuscitate them as soon as possible. Admit all for Monitoring.

HIGH ALTITUDE SICKNESS

1. **Acute Mountain Sickness (AMS)** - Nausea, Vomiting, Headache, Weakness
The best Treatment is **Descent** and Oxygen (Note that some people use Acetazolamide as prophylaxis prior to the ascent and as management but Descent is still the Best Intervention)

2. **High Altitude Cerebral Edema (HACE)** - Headache, Nausea, Vomiting, Altered Mental Status, Ataxia. Treatment: **Descent**, Oxygen, Dexamethasone

3. **High Altitude Pulmonary Edema (HAPE)** - Nausea, Vomiting, Cough, Shortness of Breath, Fever. Treatment: **Descent**, Oxygen, Nifedipine

Reminder: The best cure for all Altitude Sicknesses (AMS, HACE, HAPE) is Descent!

SUBMERSION INCIDENTS

A. Concerns and findings in these patients may include the following:
1. Trauma
2. AMS/Neurological Symptoms
3. Cardiac Arrest, Respiratory Arrest
4. Pulmonary edema
5. Vomiting
6. Abnormal vital signs (Tachycardia, Hypoxia, Apnea, etc.)
7. Dysrhythmias
8. Hypothermia

B. Management:
1. Resuscitate
2. Airway intervention
3. Full Trauma Evaluation
4. Send labs (ie. FSG, CBC, CMP, PT/PTT. Type and cross, etc.) and consider C-Spine Immobilization early on if any evidence of trauma/distracting injury or patient was drinking alcohol

TEMPERATURE RELATED ILLNESS

A. Heat

1. **Heat Exhaustion:** High Temperature and Weakness, Headache, Nausea, Vomiting. Get out of the Heat. IVF's, Cool the patient (Cooling fans, etc.)

2. **Heat Stroke:** Temperature very high - often > 104. May manifest as Alteration in Mental Status, High Temperature. Causes Multi-Organ involvement. It can cause MI, Pulmonary Complications, Renal failure, Coagulopathy and Rhabdomyolysis. Treatment: First ABC's, get out of the Heat, Rapidly Cool the body with Cool Water, Cooling Fans, IVF's. Send all labs (You may see different lab findings, including Elevated LFT's, Increased CPK, Hyponatremia, etc). Admit.

B. Cold

1. **Frostbite** - Due to Extreme Cold Temperatures at Freezing. Affects the digits mostly leading to a spectrum of numbness, redness, paleness. Management: ABC's, Take off all cold/wet clothes and Rewarm the patient Rapidly, Give Pain Medications, Tetanus Shot, Debridement, Dressing, Antibiotics, Hydration

2. **Hypothermia:** Bradycardia, Weakness, AMS, Dysrhythmias. Due to Cold Temperatures or other Etiologies (ie Endocrine Disorders, etc). Send Labs. EKG with Osborn (J) waves. Manage Airway. Immobilize C-Spine. IV, O2, Monitor. Place a Rectal Probe to Monitor the Temperature. Needs Rewarming (Remove Wet Clothes, Warm Blankets, Bair Huggers, Warm Oxygen, Warmed IV Fluids, Full Physical Examination)

RADIATION EMERGENCIES

1. **Radiation Emergencies:** Weakness, Nausea, Vomiting, Diarrhea, AMS/Confusion, Bleeding, Infection. Possible Thrombocytopenia, Neutropenia. Management: Radiation Safety Officer is in charge. Patients exposed to radiation should enter a predesignated entrance which has a separate decontamination unit so it cannot contaminate the other portions of the hospital/uncontaminated people. Radiation Detector. Wear All Protective Gear. Decontaminate the Patient by Removing and Disposing of All Contaminated Articles of Clothing, Clean Skin with Water Thoroughly. Chelating agents can be used including: Calcium Edetate, Penicillamine. Potassium Iodide are often given as well to limit the exposure to the Radioactive Iodine.

HEAD, EAR, EYE, NOSE, THROAT DISORDERS

EAR

1. Foreign Body: If safe to to remove, Remove with forceps while directly visualizing the Ear. Irrigation can be used for small items but is **Contraindicated** in anything that may swell from water (ie. vegetables). Live insects should be killed with mineral oil or 2% Lidocaine, before you remove it (Don't put anything in the ear if there is a Ruptured TM!). ENT Consult is needed for a failed attempt, an object that is unsafe to remove or a Perforated TM.

2. Labyrinthitis: Labyrinth infection. Hearing loss, Tinnitus, Vertigo. Needs Antibiotics and ENT.

3. Mastoiditis: Inflammation/Infection of the Mastoid. Pain, Swelling, Redness, Tenderness over the Mastoid. Diagnosis is Clinical and CT scan. Needs Admission, IV Antibiotics and Consult ENT

4. Ménière's Disease: Tinnitus, Vomiting, Hearing Loss. Treatment: Consider Diuretic, Antihistamine. ENT consult.

5. Otitis Media: Infection of Middle Ear. Erythema of the TM, Bulging TM. Treatment is an Antibiotic (ie Amoxicillin, Augmentin)

6. Otitis Externa: Often in Swimmers. Pain, Itch, Tender External Portion of the Ear. Redness and Swelling of the External Auditory Canal. Drainage from the ear. Treatment is Antibiotic Ear Drops (Cortisporin): Note that this is Contraindicated in patients with a Ruptured TM. If Infection of skin present as well then you can use PO Antibiotics.

7. Malignant Otitis Externa: Elderly patients, Immunocompromised patients, Diabetic patients. Diagnosis is CT scan and Stat ENT is needed. IV Antibiotics and Admission.

8. Perforated Tympanic Membrane: Pain and Loss of Hearing. Antibiotics may be given and advise the patient to keep the ear dry. Provide ENT Follow-Up.

EYE

1. **Corneal Abrasion:** Tearing, Eye Pain, Photophobia, Injected Conjunctiva. Often due to a scratch on the eye. Fluorescein (green) uptake. Give Antibiotic Ointment. Needs Ophthalmology Consult or Follow Up.

2. **Corneal Ulcer:** Occurs in contact lens users often. Tearing, Eye pain, Photophobia, Injected Conjunctiva. Fluorescein uptake of white ulcer, Slit lamp, Stat Stat Ophthalmology Consult in the ER.

3. **Purulent Endophthalmitis:** Eye pain, Blurry vision. Photophobia, Headache, Eye Discharge, Loss of vision, Eyelid Erythematous. Needs Ophthalmology Consult Stat, IV Antibiotics, Stat Ophthalmology Consult. Admit.

4. **Chalazion:** Inflammation of the Gland in the Lid. May or may not be painful. Warm Compress, Topical antibiotics. Can consider Antibiotics by mouth if any concern for concomitant infection or no improvement. If no improvement, Ophthalmology for possible incision and drainage.

5. **Hordeolum** (Stye): Bacterial Infection of the Margin of the Lid's Gland. Treatment is Warm compress and Antibacterial ointment. May consider PO Antibiotic if no improvement

6. **Acute Narrow Angle Glaucoma:** Headache, Pain in the Eye, Abdominal Pain, Nausea, Vomiting. Cloudy Cornea, Mid-Dilated Pupil, Red Conjunctiva, IOP is elevated. Stat Ophthalmology Consult. Treatment is Topical Beta Blocker (Timolol), Topical Alpha Agonist (Apraclonidine), Carbonic Anhydrase Inhibitor (Acetazolamide) IV/PO, Mannitol IV, Check IOP each hour. Topical Pilocarpine and Stat Ophthalmology Evaluation in the ER and Admission

7. **Hyphema:** Blood in Anterior Chamber. Keep the Patient Sitting Up. Ophthalmology consult Stat. Should Admit due to many potential complications (such as Rebleeding, Vision Loss, Elevation of Intraocular Pressure and the increased chance of acute narrow angle glaucoma, etc). Often occurs in Trauma but not always. Ensure that it is not due to a Globe Rupture, which would have a Positive Siedel Test. Do not test for IOP until you have excluded a Globe Rupture! Make sure Ophthalmology is Consulted Stat. Admit.

8. **Hypopyon:** Collection of Pus/WBC's in the Anterior Chamber of the eye. Often due to another disorder that needs to be addressed/managed.

9. **Retrobulbar Hematoma:** Due to Trauma. Pain, Proptosis, Possible Mild Visual Loss. Diagnosis is CT Orbit. Emergent Ophthalmology consult for Lateral Canthotomy

10. **Iritis:** Blurry vision, Eye pain, Photophobia, Injected Conjunctiva. Worsened visual acuity than usual. Dx: Slit Lamp with Cells and Flare. Needs Ophthalmology Consult. Must figure out the Underlying Etiology of the Iritis

11. **Retinal Detachment:** Flashing lights, Curtain coming down over eye, Floaters, Decreased vision. Diagnosis: Ultrasound. Ophthalmology Consult Stat. Admit.

12. **Retinal Vascular Occlusion:**

12a. **CRAO:** Due to Embolus, Thrombus, etc. Painless loss of vision. On Ocular examination, you may find "Cherry Red Spot" and Retinal Pallor. Treatment is Ocular Massage for 15 seconds and Ophthalmology Consult Stat. Admit.

12b. **CRVO:** Thrombus. Loss of vision, Painless. Fundoscopy: "Blood and Thunder", Hemorrhage on Fundoscopic Exam. Stat Ophthalmology Consult Stat

13. Cellulitis

13a. **Preseptal Cellulitis (Periorbital Cellulitis):** Warm, Swollen, Erythematous Eyelid. Diagnosis: CT Orbit. Needs Oral Antibiotic (ie. Augmentin). If Toxic in appearance, needs IV Antibiotic, Ophthalmology Consult and Admission

13b. **Postseptal Cellulitis (Orbital Cellulitis):** Warm, Swollen, Erythematous Eyelid and Proptosis, Ophthalmoplegia (limited or painful or no EOMs). Decreased vision, Diagnosis: CT orbit. Needs Ophthalmology Consult Stat, IV Antibiotics

14. **Blepharitis:** Inflammation of the region where the eyelid and eyelash join. "Crusting" along the margin of the eyelid. Pruritic, Erythematous, Swollen Region of Eyelid, near the Eyelashes. Management is Antibiotics, Warm Compresses

15. **Conjunctivitis:** Bacterial Conjunctivitis: Tearing, Discharge (Purulent), Injected Conjunctiva. Management is Antibacterial Eyedrops. If you can't distinguish viral conjunctivitis from bacterial, empirically treat as though bacterial. A very dangerous form of Conjunctivitis is due to Gonorrhea. It causes Heavy Purulent Discharge. This needs IV Antibiotics and Antibiotic Eyedrops. Needs Stat Ophthalmology Consult.

16. **Dacrocystitis:** Swelling, Erythema and Tenderness over the Region of the Lacrimal Sac, due to blockage of the Nasolacrimal Duct. Tearing. Management is Antibiotics, Ophthalmology Consult

17. **Chemical Burn to the Eye:** Needs Immediate Irrigation of the Eyes with Sterile NS. Needs pH measurements to ensure that the pH is normalizing and stays normal. Consult Ophthalmology

18. **Eye Foreign Body:** As long as there are No Contraindications, Corneal Foreign Bodies are Removed with either a cotton swab or with a 25 gauge needle, very carefully. Ensure that patient doesn't have a Ruptured Globe after the procedure.

Ophthalmology Appointment for FB (ie. Removal of Rust Ring) should be done either the same day or the next day or Ophthalmology ER consult.

19. **Optic Neuritis:** Often a Manifestation in those with Multiple Sclerosis. Eye pain, Visual loss, Partial Loss of Color Vision. Needs Ophthalmology Consultation. If concerned for MS, Consult Neurology as well. Needs IV Steroids. Admit.

CEREBRAL VENOUS SINUS THROMBOSIS

1. **Cavernous Sinus Thrombosis:** Headache, Neck pain, Fever, Chemosis, Ophthalmoplegia, Ptosis, Periorbital Edema, Cranial Nerve Palsy, Proptosis, Loss of some Visual Acuity. Diagnosis: CT scan. Consult: Surgery. Treatment is IV Antibiotics. Possible Role of Anticoagulation in Management has been shown in some research but it is Not conclusive. ICU admission. Neurology, Ophthalmology Consultation Stat. Admit.

NOSE

1. **Epistaxis:** Anterior or Posterior (Posterior has more complications and needs Admission). Ask patient to blow nose to get clots out. Direct External Pressure. If you see an **Anterior Bleed** and Direct pressure x 15 minutes doesn't work, try a Silver Nitrate Stick. If neither of these work, try Anterior Nasal Packing. If this still doesn't work, get an ENT Consult and give Antibiotics.

2. **Posterior Epistaxis** Needs Posterior Nasal Packing, Antibiotics, ENT consult and Hospital Admission due to Higher Risk of Complications.

3. **Reminder:** Note that **Anyone with Any type of Nasal Packing needs Antibiotics** (ie. Augmentin) to Prevent Toxic Shock Syndrome.

4. **Foreign Body:** Foul smelling Rhinorrhea, Possible Unilateral Nosebleed, One nose obstructed. Often in children. Remove FB with Suction or Positive Pressure. ENT consult if unable

5. **Sinusitis:** Nasal congestion, Pain in the Face, Fever, Sinus pressure, Headache, Rhinorrhea, Tender Sinus Palpation. Management is a Case-dependent Clinical Decision on Antibiotics (ie. Augmentin) versus Supportive care initially for a few days in mild cases, to watch for improvement.

6. **Nasal Fracture:** Tenderness of the Nose, Swollen. Look for a Septal Hematoma. If a Septal Hematoma present, the Treatment is Incision and Drainage and Ice, Pain Medications, Decongestants, Anterior Nasal Packing, Antibiotics, ENT

Note: An untreated Septal Hematoma causes Avascular Necrosis

OROPHARYNX/THROAT

1. **Ludwig's Angina:** Infection of the submandibular region/bottom of mouth's soft tissue that manifests with pain and swelling and that can lead to a loss of the airway. Painful, Swelling, Airway Management. Needs IV Antibiotics, IVF's and Stat ENT/Surgery Consult. ICU Admit.

2. **Sialolithiasis:** Stone in the Salivary duct. Diagnosis is Clinical. Give Sialogogue to help pass the stone, Massage the Gland (if does not work, ENT consult). Give Antibiotics to treat any concomitant infection. ENT Follow Up.

3. **Epiglottitis:** Inflammation, Infection of Epiglottis, Strawberry like in appearance. Hyperextended Neck, Patient sits forward. Prepare for Airway Management Stat by Expert. Let the Patient stay in a Comfortable Position. Lateral Neck X-ray: Thumbprint sign. IV Antibiotics. Stat ENT, Anesthesia. ICU Admit.

4. **Tracheitis:** Respiratory Distress, Secretions. Airway, Antibiotics

5. **Peritonsillar Abscess:** Peritonsillar Infection, Peritonsillar region with Abscess, Sore throat, Fever, Drooling, Hoarseness, Muffled voice, Painful swallowing, Difficulty swallowing, Ear pain, Deviated Uvula in the opposite direction of the Peritonsillar abscess. Diagnosis Clinical. Treatment: Needle Aspiration by ENT and Antibiotics

6. **Pharyngitis/Tonsillitis:** Sore throat, Fever, Lymph Nodes. Diagnosis: Clinical (Centor Criteria: No Cough, Fever, Pharyngeal Erythema or Tonsillar Exudate, Anterior Cervical Lymphadenopathy), Rapid Strep, Throat Culture. Treatment: If Strep Pharyngitis: Antibiotic (Penicillin: Bicillin or Amoxicillin). Note that Giving Antibiotics in a timely fashion for Strep Pharyngitis can prevent Rheumatic fever but not necessarily Glomerulonephritis.

7. **Infectious Mononucleosis (IM)** should be kept in the Differential of Pharyngitis. Use the Monospot test to diagnose IM. IM presents with Posterior Cervical Lymph Nodes, Fever, Extreme Fatigue and a Sore Throat. Management is Supportive treatment. Crucial Point: No Contact Sports because Splenic Rupture is possible in these patients. Some patients with Infectious Mono who have been misdiagnosed with Strep and treated with Amoxicillin may return with a Rash.

8. **Retropharyngeal Abscess:** Abscess in Retropharyngeal region. Presents with a Sore throat, Hoarseness, Fever, Neck pain, Difficulty swallowing, Voice changes,

Difficulty with extending the neck, may feel a neck mass (abscess), Respiratory Distress, Drooling, Hoarse voice, Throat pain, Neck pain. Diagnosis is a Lateral X-ray of Soft tissue of Neck (which may show Widening of the Retropharyngeal space) or a CT Soft Tissue Neck. Management: Manage Airway. ENT Stat Consult for Possible OR Drainage, IV Antibiotics (Broad Spectrum), IV Fluids, Admit

HEMATOLOGY & ONCOLOGY DISORDERS

1. Blood Transfusion

1. Complications: Acute Hemolytic Reaction, Delayed Hemolytic Reaction, Hypersensitivity/Allergic reaction, Infections, Fever. The Initial Management for all of these is to Stop the transfusion.

2. Hemostatic Disorders

1. **Hemophilia A:** Factor 8 Deficiency. Hematuria, Bruising, Hematoma, Hemarthrosis, Hemorrhage, Intracranial Hemorrhage. Always have a low index of suspicion for a Bleed in these patients, even after a minor trauma. Labs: Increased PTT. Treatment is Factor VIII Replacement, Desmopressin

2. **DIC:** Various Pathologies, Infections, trauma, bites are only a few etiologies of DIC. Manifests with hemorrhage, thrombosis. Labs will show Increased Fibrin Split Products, Decreased Fibrinogen, Low Platelets, Increased PT/PTT. Schistocytes Present. Management is mainly to Treat the Underlying Etiology. Also must manage the Symptoms of Presentation.

3. **Thrombocytopenia:** Decreased Platelets. May present with Bleeding. May present with Rash (Petechiae). Can be secondary to Medications, Infections, Disorders (ie. TTP, etc.)

4. **Heparin Induced Thrombocytopenia (HIT):** Can occur in those on Heparin, leading to Thrombocytopenia. Management is to Stop the Heparin (and substitute with a Direct Thrombin Inhibitor, such as Argatroban)

5. **ITP:** Thrombocytopenia. May be secondary to virus. Autoimmune. In children, supportive treatment and in adults the management is steroids. In symptomatic adults, give steroids. If symptoms are present, Admit.

6. **Von Willebrand Disease:** Platelet cannot adhere due to either Decreased, Damaged or Absent VWF. Causes Bleeding. Increased PTT, Increased Bleeding Time. Treatment is Desmopressin.

7. **HUS, TTP:** See Oral Boards Review Section for Description and Mnemonics

3. Red Blood Cell Disorder

1. Anemia

   A. **Hemoglobinopathies**

      a. **Sickle Cell Disease:** A Hereditary Disorder that results from the Sickling of RBC's due to Abnormal Hemoglobin (Hgb S). May Present with Pain Crises, Splenic Sequestration, Dactylitis, Bone Pain, Aplastic Crisis, Osteomyelitis, Avascular Necrosis, Acute Chest Syndrome, Priapism, CVA, Infections. Management: IV Hydration, Oxygen, Pain Medications and in certain circumstances, Need Exchange Transfusion (ie Acute Chest Syndrome, Priapism, CVA). Specialty Consultation with Hematology. See Oral Boards Section.

   B. **Hypochromic**

      a. **Iron Deficiency:** Often times secondary to heavy blood loss (ie menstrual periods). May also be due to Malignancy, Various Disorders, Inadequate Intake, Medications, etc. Treatment is Ferrous Sulfate, Managing and Correcting the Underlying Precipitant

   C. **Hemolytic** —> Thalassemias, Hereditary Spherocytosis, G6PDH deficiency...
      a. G6PDH Deficiency: Often due to Medications and Infections. Management is to Avoid these Medications (ie. Sulfa)
      b. Hereditary Spherocytosis: RBC has an abnormal shape that leads to it getting destroyed in the Spleen. Needs a Splenectomy.
      c. Thalassemia: Due to problematic globin chains. These patients have Anemia, increased risk of infection and get transfused a lot (iron overload is a risky complication in these patients due to their multiple transfusions).

   D. **Aplastic Anemia** —>Pancytopenia (Decreased ability to make RBC, WBC, Platelets) = Anemia, Leukopenia, Thrombocytopenia, Causing Pallor, Malaise, Pain, Bruising, Bleeding etc.

   E. **Megaloblastic** —> Vitamin B12 deficiency (Pernicious Anemia, Vegetarians), Folate deficiency (Alcoholism, Pregnancy, Elderly). Management is giving either B12, Folate in the patients with the deficiency and treat/manage the underlying cause

2. **Methemoglobinemia:** Possible symptoms: Cyanotic, Dysrhythmia, Chest Pain, SOB, AMS, Headache. Management: Oxygen, Methylene blue

4. White Blood Cell Disorders

A. Leukemias
A. Thrombocytopenia, Anemia, Leukopenia, Lymphadenopathy, Lethargy, Pain, Weight loss, Fever, Infection, Bleeding. Acute leukemias are dangerous with the formation of blast cells. Needs Immediate Hospitalization for Management, Oncology Consult. If Neutropenic Fever, Send Cultures, Give Antibiotics. Types of acute leukemia: AML and ALL. Chronic leukemias include: CML and CLL. Diagnosis is Bone Marrow Biopsy. All of these need Admission and Oncology Consultation

B. **Multiple myeloma:** Plasma Cell Neoplastic Proliferation, Bone Pain, Hypercalcemia, Anemia, Renal Failure. Infections, Bone discomfort (Back pain). Diagnosis: SPEP and free light chain assay. Treatment: Chemotherapy

C. **Leukopenia:** Low WBCs. Causes: Infection, Medications, Endocrine disorders, Cancer, Aplastic Anemia, Toxins, Radiation. Treatment is treating the underlying cause

5. Lymphoma

a. **Hodgkin Lymphoma:** Painless Lymphadenopathy, Fever, Weight Loss. Diagnosis is Lymph Node Biopsy. Treatment is Chemotherapy and Radiation

b. **Non-Hodgkin Lymphoma:** Painless Lymphadenopathy. Diagnosis is Lymph node Biopsy. Treatment is Chemotherapy and Radiation

6. **Neutropenic Fever:** This is an Oncologic Emergency. Send all Labs (CBC, CMP, etc), Blood Cultures, Urinalysis, Urine Culture, Do CXR, Send Cultures from any catheter sites, etc. Do additional tests per symptoms of the patient (ie. CT Head and LP if concern for Meningitis). Do a thorough physical exam. ANC <500. Scenario: Chemo patient with a Fever and a Low WBC, Low ANC. Must start IV Antibiotics. Place the patient on Reverse Isolation. Admit.

7. **Tumor Lysis Syndrome:** Occurs in Chemotherapy patients —> Cells die —> Increased Uric Acid, Increased Phosphate, Increased Potassium. Can cause Renal Failure and Low Calcium. Treatment is Electrolyte Correction and IV Fluids.

8. **Superior Vena Cava Obstruction:** Shortness of Breath, Swelling of Body, Face in patients with Malignancy (often Lung Ca). Diagnosis: CT scan. Management: Steroids, Oncology Consultation Stat, Radiation.

9. **Hypercalcemia:** AMS, N/V, Fatigue, Back Pain. Tx: IV Fluids (NS), Diuretics, etc.

IMMUNOLOGY

COLLAGEN VASCULAR DISEASE

1. **Reiter's Syndrome:** Arthritis, Urethritis, Conjunctivitis. Management is Antibiotics and Pain Medications.

2. **Raynaud's:** Vasospasm of the Digits causing Coldness, Paresthesias, etc. Avoid the Cold. Warm the region. It should resolve. If it doesn't always ensure that there is good arterial supply immediately (and that there isn't a more serious underlying etiology).

3. **Scleroderma:** It can either be Localized or Systemic. The Skin Thickens due to too much collagen and calcium deposition and so do various other organs in the body [ie. the GI tract (ie. esophagus)]. It can also cause issues with the Kidneys and Lungs. In the systemic form one may also have generalized symptoms such as Weakness, etc. Skin Thickening that affects Multiple Organs (Skin, GI tract, Kidneys, Lungs)

4. **Rheumatoid Arthritis:** Arthritis of Multiple joints. + Rheumatoid Factor. Rheumatoid Nodules. May have Generalized Weakness. Management: Pain Medications and Corticosteroids or Sulfasalazine.

5. **Systemic Lupus Erythematosus**
   a) Autoimmune disorder which may manifest in various Organ Systems (Cardiac, Pulmonary, Dermatological, ENT, Neurological, Renal, Rheumatologic). May present with Arthralgias, Fever, Butterfly rash, CNS involved, Renal, Photosensitivity, Pleuritis, Pericarditis, Oral Ulcers. Diagnosis: Possible + ANA, Anemia, Thrombocytopenia. Treatment: Steroids, Salicylates, Nsaids, etc.

6. Vasculitis

   a) **Temporal Arteritis:** Vasculitis. Can cause blindness if untreated. Headache, Pain along side of scalp, PMR (Jaw Claudication, Malaise/Weakness), Fever, ESR Elevated (ESR >50). If you think it's Temporal Arteritis start steroids immediately and get a Ophthalmology Consultation Stat. Temporal Artery Biopsy is Confirmative but Start Steroids before this if you suspect it. If untreated, this can lead to blindness.

   b) **Takayasu Arteritis:** Vasculitis that is more common in women. Malaise, Fever, Muscle aches, Joint aches. Can cause a loss of or a diminished pulse in the arms or legs. Management is Steroids. In cases that are more severe with diminished arterial blood supply, the patient may need vascular surgery intervention.

HYPERSENSITIVITY

1. **Allergic Reaction:** A Hypersensitivity reaction to something (ie. food, medication, etc.) that can manifest with different symptoms (ie. hives)

2. **Anaphylaxis:** Allergic reaction to something (ie food, material, medication, etc. but often times due to an unknown etiology). Dyspnea, Swelling, Nausea, Vomiting, Diarrhea, Skin Rash, Flushed, Itchy, Wheezing, Hives, Abdominal Pain, Syncope, Hypotension, Stridor, Runny nose, Cough. Can present with Practically any Organ System. Skin issue, Respiratory issue, Hypotension are some ways it may manifest. Treatment for Anaphylaxis: Epinephrine first. Epinephrine (IM) especially if patient has respiratory distress, airway edema or is hypotensive. Be very careful and reconsider using this in anyone with known heart disease/issues or is Elderly. Oxygen, IVF's (NS), Epinephrine, Steroids, Benadryl, Ranitidine. Keep in mind that in a patient on Beta blockers, Epinephrine may not work, so if unsuccessful, use Glucagon. Disposition - ICU

Mild allergic reaction: Benadryl, Ranitidine, Steroids, Observation for at least 4 to 8 hours in the ER. May be able to discharge a very mild allergic reaction if improvement is clear (resolution of symptoms and no rebound), after many hours of Observation and No use of epinephrine was needed. If surely safe to discharge, then ensure that the patient receives Epipen, Steroids, Benadryl and Immediate Allergist follow up with strict follow up an instructions for same day or early the next day.

3. **Angioedema** - Either due to C1 esterase deficiency or ACE inhibitor medication. Consider Early Intubation for Oral Edema. Admit. FFP is given for C1 Esterase Deficiency generally.

TRANSPLANT RELATED PROBLEMS

1. Patients with Transplants are placed on Immunosuppressants to help keep the Transplant Intact and Attempt to Prevent Rejection. However, Immunosuppressants in turn can Increase the Risk of Infection in these patients. Therefore, in Transplant Patients, you must consider: Rejection, Infection, Toxicity from Immunosuppressants.

2. **Infection:** ie CMV, Herpes, Bacterial etc. Need to be treated with appropriate agents (ie. Antibiotics, Antivirals, etc).

3. **Rejection:** Tenderness over the Graft, Malaise, Abnormal labs, Pain (ie. Heart Transplant: Chest Pain, SOB, Dysrhythmias, CHF) (ie. Liver Transplant: Abdominal Pain, Fever), (ie. Renal Transplant: Edema, HTN, Oliguria). Management is Steroids (Solumedrol) and if evidence of infection, Antibiotics

IMMUNE COMPLEX DISORDERS

1. Kawasaki syndrome
   Kawasaki
   1. **Mnemonic: CHECK**
   2. **CHECK Mnemonic: C**onjunctivitis, **C**ardiac complications, **C**ervical Lymphadenopathy, **C**racked Lips, **H**eart complications, **E**dematous Hands/Feet, **E**rythematous Hands/Feet, **E**rythematous Mouth/Lips, **K**awasaki
   3. Can affect the mucous membranes, heart, skin, lymph nodes, brain, joints, etc.
   4. Worst Complication: Coronary Artery Aneurysm, Sudden Cardiac Death
   5. Fever for at least 5 days must be present, along with at least Four of any of the following: Conjunctivitis bilaterally, lymphadenopathy in cervical region (neck), rash, strawberry tongue, lips cracked, erythematous mouth and lips, erythematous hands/feet, edematous hands/feet, desquamation
   6. Treatment: IVIG, Aspirin, Cardiology Consultation, Admit,
   7. **CHECK Mnemonic: C**onjunctivitis, **C**ardiac complications, **C**ervical Lymphadenopathy, **C**racked Lips, **H**eart complications, **E**dematous hands/feet, **E**rythematous hands/feet, **E**rythematous Mouth/Lips, **K**awasaki

2. Rheumatic Fever: Can occur secondary to Strep Pharyngitis. Pericarditis, Polyarthritis, Choreic movements, Skin Nodules, Erythema Marginatum. May also have Fever, Joint aches. Management is Antibiotics

3. Sarcoidosis: May manifest with Weakness, Cough, Erythema Nodosum, Dyspnea, etc or May be entirely Asymptomatic. Can affect many different organ systems (Cardiac, Pulmonary, Ocular, Dermatological, Lymph Nodes, Rheumatological). Management: Steroids

4. Post-Streptococcal Glomerulonephritis: Can occur after Strep Pharyngitis. Hematuria, HTN, Edema. Management: Antibiotics

INFECTIOUS DISEASES

BACTERIAL

1. **Botulism:** Due to a Neurotoxin. Weakness, Respiratory issues, Constipation. Infants may have Poor Feeding and a Cry that is Not strong, Weakness. Management: Airway Management, Antitoxin.

2. **Chlamydia:** Abdominal Pain, Vaginal discharge. Can be Asymptomatic in men. May manifest as PID or in other manners. Treat with Antibiotics that covers both Chlamydia and Gonorrhea (and Trichomonas) as they often travel together.

3. **Gonococcus:** Abdominal Pain, Vaginal Discharge. Can be Asymptomatic in men. May manifest as PID. Treat with Antibiotics. Can also manifest as Arthritis, Tenosynovitis. Send Cultures (Throat, Rectal, Cervical). If Septic Arthritis, Arthrocentesis is needed. Note that Disseminated Gonococcal infection can occur. May present with Tender Pustules on the Skin. May present with Septic Arthritis. May present with Sepsis. May Present with Tenosynovitis. Needs IV Antibiotics and Admission. Treat with Antibiotics that covers both Chlamydia and Gonorrhea (and Trichomonas) as they often travel together. Note that Neonates can also present with Gonococcal infection from the mother, by presenting with Conjunctivitis. Also needs Antibiotics and Admission.

4. **Meningococcus:** Fever, AMS, Seizure, Nausea, Vomiting, Headache, Neck Stiffness, Rash. Needs Immediate Isolation. Send Labs (CBC with Differential, CMP, PT/PTT, Blood Cultures). Bacterial Meningitis needs Antibiotics and Steroids. Needs IV fluids. Needs CT Head (if any concern for a Mass Lesion: ie Papilledema, Focal Neurological Deficits, Immunocompromised, etc.) and a Lumbar Puncture (Send CSF studies i.e. Cell Count, Glucose, Protein, Gram stain, Culture), if stable and No Contraindications. Place the Patient in Respiratory Isolation.

5. **Mycobacteria:**
a) **Tuberculosis:**
b) Primary TB (Asymptomatic). Latent TB (Asymptomatic). Active TB (Lungs: Night Sweats, Cough, Weight Loss, Blood in Cough) (Bones = Potts disease) (CNS: TB Meningitis) (Lymph Nodes)
b) PPD is the test to see if a patient was exposed (Latent infection)
c) Latent TB: Management is 9 months of Isoniazid (INH)
d) Active TB: Rifampin, INH, Ethambutol, Pyrazinamide **(Mnemonic: RIPE)**

6. **Gas Gangrene:** Gas forming organisms, like Anaerobes lead to infection (ie Clostridium Perfingens). Leads to Necrosis, Gangrene. Needs Stat Surgery Consultation for Surgical Debridement, IV Antibiotics, IV Fluids, OR.

7. Sepsis/Bacteremia

a) **Systemic Inflammatory Response - Criteria for SIRS:** Tachycardia (HR >90), Fever/Hypothermia (Temp >38C or <36C), Leukocytosis (WBC >12) or Leukopenia (WBC <4) or >10% Bands and Tachypnea (RR >20 or PaCO2 <32)

b) **Sepsis:** SIRS + Source of Infection

c) **Septic Shock:** Sepsis + End Organ Damage, Hypotension

8. Toxic Shock Syndrome: Presents with Hypotension, Fever, Rash (Macular, Erythroderma, Desquamation), GI, CNS, Renal, etc. Possible Etiology: Tampon, Packing or any Foreign Body left in a person. Treatment: IV Antibiotics, IV Fluids, Removal of the Foreign Body (ie Removal of the Tampon)

9. Syphilis: Primary is a Painless Chancre, Secondary is with Maculopapular rash, Lymphadenopathy. Tertiary is Neurological and Cardiac issues. Treatment is Penicillin

10. Tetanus: Rigidity, Trismus, Spasms, Respiratory Distress. Give Tetanus Immune Globulin, Antibiotics, Lorazepam

BIOLOGICAL WARFARE AGENTS

1. Sarin, VX: Block Acetylcholinesterase Leading to Increased ACh (Cholinergic): Vomiting, Diarrhea, Lacrimation, Urinary Frequency, AMS. Treatment: Atropine, Pralidoxime

2. Tularemia: Lymphadenopathy, Ulcers on the Skin are possible

3. Plague: Buboes (Tender Lymph Nodes, Large), Fever/Chills, Sepsis

4. Anthrax:
Cutaneous: Eschar on the Skin, Edematous
Pulmonary (Inhalational) - Respiratory Distress, Pleural Effusion
GI - GI Bleed, Abdominal Pain

5. Smallpox: Pustules all over the body present with the same in appearance

FUNGAL

Pneumocystis Carinii: Always consider this in HIV patients as a cause of Pneumonia. Fever and Cough. In addition to covering for CAP, with Ceftriaxone and Azithromycin, these patients also need Bactrim and also need Steroids if the A-a Gradient is >35 or the PaO2 is <70. CXR shows Diffuse Interstitial Infiltrates. Admit.

PROTOZOAN/PARASITES

1. **Malaria:** High Fever/Chills, Nausea, Vomiting. May be Anemic. Management depends on the susceptibility and resistance pattern in the Endemic region (ie. Quinine, Mefloquine, Atovaquone-Proguanil)

2. **Toxoplasmosis:** Headache, AMS, Seizure, Neurological Symptoms/Deficits. Often occurs in patients with HIV. Diagnosis: CT Head may show Ring Lesion. Management: Pyrimethamine, Sulfadiazine

TICK BORNE

1. **Ehrlichiosis:** The Tick is the vector that spreads this. May cause Fatigue, Rash. Thrombocytopenia, Leukopenia. Treatment is Doxycycline. Complications include Possible Neurological/Cardiological/Renal/Respiratory issues

2. **Lyme Disease:** Rash, Weakness, Fever, Erythema Migrans. Target Lesion. Could have Cardiological or Neurological Complications later (ie Meningitis, AV blocks). Management is Doxycycline for the Rash. Can consider Ceftriaxone when Cardiac or Neurological Complications are also present.

3. **Rocky Mountain Spotted Fever:** Recent visit to area with possible ticks. Fever, Headache, Rash (Rash starts on wrists, ankles and then spreads to the trunk, palms and soles), Nausea, Vomiting, Fatigue, Muscle Aches, Nausea, Conjunctivitis. Treatment: Doxycycline

VIRAL

1. **Infectious Mononucleosis:** Due to EBV. Sore throat, Fever, Lethargy/Malaise, Posterior Cervical Lymphadenopathy. Dx: Positive Monospot test. Supportive Treatment. Warn the patient: No Contact Sports because the patient can have Splenomegaly and Sports/Trauma can lead to Splenic Rupture.

2. **Influenza:** Fatigue, Cough, Muscle aches, Fever, Pharyngitis, Rhinorrhea. Influenza Test. Treat with Antiviral (ie. Tamiflu) if the symptoms lasted <48 hours. Patients over the age of 65, Those in the Medical field, Immunocompromised

Patients and Children should get the Influenza vaccination yearly.

3. **Hantavirus:** Often due to the Exposure to Urine/Other Secretions from Mice. Fatigue, Thrombocytopenia, Fluid overload in the Lungs. Management is Supportive.

4. **Herpes Simplex:** See Dermatology section

5. **Herpes Zoster:** Shingles: Rash along a Single Dermatome (Can be Multidermatomal in Immunocompromised Patients). Management is Acyclovir/ Valacyclovir.

6. **Herpes Zoster Ophthalmicus:** Vesicles along the Trigeminal Nerve Region. Consult Ophthalmology Stat. Give Acyclovir or Valacyclovir. Note: In a Herpes patient with a Vesicle on the Tip of the Nose, Always Examine the Eyes (Slit lamp shows Dendritic Lesions).

7. **Varicella:** Chickenpox. Lesions are in different stages.

8. **Rabies:** Pain at the region of the bite. Fatigue, AMS, Aggravation, Spasms are Symptoms of Actual Rabies. Those at High risk of Rabies Exposure should be Pre-Vaccinated. Those with Possible Post-Exposure, should also be given the vaccination as soon as possible, on subsequent visits (ie. day 0, day 3, day 7, day 14, etc). Give it Prior to symptom onset, after which chance of survival are significantly lower.

RHEUMATOLOGY/MUSCULOSKELETAL

1. **Osteomyelitis:** Inflammation, Infection of the Bone. Give IV Antibiotics. Diagnosed with Xray, CT or MRI or Bone Scan. Needs Orthopedic Consult. Admission.

2. **Septic Arthritis:** Fever, Warm, Tender, Red Joint, Painful, Diagnosis is Arthrocentesis (May have Positive Gram Stain, Elevated WBC count often >50,000). Management: Stat Orthopedic Consult, IV Antibiotics. Admit

3. **Crystal Arthropathies**

a. **Gout:** Painful Joint, Warm, Often Big Toe involved (Podagra). Top possible. Diagnosis: Arthrocentesis: Negatively Birefringent. Uric Acid Crystals in Synovial Fluid. Tx: Nsaid

b. **Pseudogout:** Painful Joint. Diagnosis: Arthrocentesis. Positively Birefringent, Calcium Pyrophosphate Crystals in the Synovial Fluid. Tx is Nsaid

4. **Rheumatoid Arthritis:** A disorder that can cause Fatigue, Loss of weight and Affect the Joints (Arthritis), Skin, Lungs, Brain, Heart and Kidneys

5. **Osteoarthritis:** Arthritis that occurs more often in the Elderly. Causes Joint Pain

6. **Congenital Dislocation of the Hip (Developmental Dysplasia of the Hip):** This is an abnormality often found in infants/children in which there is a developmental deformity of either the Hip joint or the Femur fitting into it, leading to lack of appropriate anatomical contact between the two. Causes Limp, Leg Length Discrepancy, Skin Fold on Thigh Abnormality. Management is dependent on the child's age. Harness vs. Reduction vs Surgical Management are generally the choices.

7. **Rhabdomyolysis:** Muscle Breakdown, Muscle Weakness, Urine Dark, Muscles aches, Weakness. CPK is high. Complications are Hyperkalemia, Acute Renal Failure. Often caused by Excessive Muscle Use, Trauma, Drugs, Lightning Injury, Prolonged Immobilization, Compartment Syndrome. May have Myoglobinuria. Send CBC, CPK, CMP. Urinalysis. Do EKG. May see Hyperkalemia. Treat it. Treatment is Hydrating the patient with IVF's (NS). Admit. In a patient with Renal Failure, Nephrology Consultation is needed for Possible Dialysis.

8. **Bursitis:** Inflamed Bursa characterized by Edema and Pain over a Joint region. Need to Elevate it and Place Ice

9. **Carpal Tunnel Syndrome:** Median Nerve is Compressed. Leads to Numbness and Tingling (Paresthesias) over the Region of the Hand that the Median Nerve supplies. Occurs most often in those who use their hands (ie. in those who type a lot). Management is to Place a Volar Splint, Possible Steroid Injections, Pain Medications and Follow Up. For cases that these are not beneficial, Surgical intervention may be considered.

10. **Felon:** Infection in the Pulp of the Fingertip. Needs Incision and Drainage and Antibiotics.

11. **Paronychia:** Infection on the Side of the Nail Fold which Needs Drainage if pus is present using a scalpel providing there are no contraindications. Antibiotics. If No pus, Consider Warm Compress, Antibiotics. Wound Check in 12 hrs or immediately if worsening.

12. **Flexor Tenosynovitis:** A Very Painful, Flexed Digit, Very Painful with Passive Extension, Swollen Finger, Tender Finger over Flexor Tendon Sheath
Needs IV Antibiotics and a Stat Hand Surgeon/Orthopedic Consult and Admit

13. **Herpetic Whitlow:** Infection of the Fingertip with Vesicle(s) due to Herpes virus. Do **not** drain this! Elevate it and cover with Dry gauze. May give Acyclovir. Often seen in Healthcare Workers

NEUROLOGY

CRANIAL NERVE DISORDERS

1. **Idiopathic Facial Nerve Paralysis (Bell's Palsy)** - Facial Droop Unilaterally. Bell's Palsy has **No** sparing of the forehead. Therefore when you ask the patient to raise their eyebrow, they will Not be able to for the most part. However, be wary of your diagnosis - Make sure you're not Missing a Stroke (A Stroke generally Spares the Forehead)! Management of Bell's Palsy is an Antiviral (ie. Acyclovir), Steroid

DEMYELINATING DISORDERS

1. **Multiple Sclerosis** - Sensory, Motor, Visual, Urinary Changes. "Remitting and Relapsing". Neurological Symptoms Separated by "Space and Time". Acute Exacerbations. Diagnosis: MRI. Neurology Consult. Need IV Steroids

HEADACHE

1. **Migraine** - Phonophobia, Headache, Light Sensitivity, Nausea, Vomiting (Detrimental Differential: Subarachnoid Hemorrhage presents with the same symptoms, so be careful with your diagnosis!)

2. **Cluster** - Rhinorrhea, Lacrimation. Retro-orbital Pain, Headaches. Injected Conjunctiva. Episodes are spaced out weeks apart at a time. Always Consider More Serious Causes on the Differential

INFECTIONS/INFLAMMATORY DISORDERS

1. **Encephalitis:** Inflamed Brain. Headache, Seizure, AMS, Fever. Do CT Head, Lumbar Puncture. Management: Antibiotics, Steroids and if Viral, Antiviral (ie. in instances of HSV Encephalitis). Admit

2. **Meningitis:** Infection of the Meninges. Headache, Neck Stiffness, Nausea, Vomiting, Fever/Chills. Photophobia. Bacterial - Dangerous. Needs Labs, Cultures, CT Head, Lumbar puncture (CSF studies). IV Steroids, IV Antibiotics. Admission.

NEUROMUSCULAR DISORDERS

1. **Guillain-Barré Syndrome** - Peripheral Demyelination. May occur after a viral illness (ie Diarrhea caused by a virus). Ascending Weakness, Loss of Reflexes,

Possible Respiratory Compromise. Neurology Consultation. Management: Assess Airway. Order CT Head, Labs (CBC, CMP), Urinalysis, Lumbar Puncture. Management: Airway, IVIG, Plasmapheresis. ICU admission

2. **Myasthenia Gravis** - Autoimmune. Weakness, Visual issues (Diplopia), Ptosis. Worse with increased use. May cause Respiratory Distress. Send Labs, Toxicological studies, Urinalysis, CT Head. Neurology Consultation. Management: Airway, Pyridostigmine or Neostigmine. Note: If intubating these patients, **Never** give paralytics because they have a prolonged action in these patients (Don't give succinylcholine, it is contraindicated). ICU admission

OTHER CONDITIONS OF THE BRAIN

1. **Parkinson's Disease:** Neurogenerative disorder that is characterized by Bradykinesia, Resting tremor, Rigidity, Constipation, Posture Instability. Treatments: Levodopa, Ropnirole, Pramipexole.

2. **Pseudotumor Cerebri:** Visual changes, Headache, Papilledema. CT Head, LP. Management: Some Pressure alleviated with LP. Acetazolamide.

SEIZURE DISORDERS

1. **Febrile Seizure** -
    A. **Simple Febrile Seizure:** Lasts <15 minutes and only occurs one time in 24 hours. Child is age 6 months old to 5 years old with a Fever and a Seizure who is Nontoxic appearing and Nonfocal. Seizure is Generalized. If the child is under 12 months old, always consider a Lumbar Puncture and Labs, Imaging, etc. (and also as a precautionary measure in those under 18 months). If older than this and well appearing, happy, playful, and fitting of all the criteria above, may consider finding the cause of the fever (UA, etc.) and ensuring proper parent follow up, education.

    B. **Complex Febrile Seizure:** Lasts >15 minutes, recurs more than one time in 24 hours. Child is not within age bracket listed above. Nontoxic. Seizure may be Focal. Needs a Full workup, including Labs/Testing (CBC, UA, Blood culture, Urine culture, Lumbar puncture, CSF studies). If ill appearing, needs Admission. If well appearing, can consider d/c but with very close follow up (return in 12 hours or immediately for any concerning changes). Always keep in mind that these patients can have Bacterial Meningitis, so Any concern needs Admission!

2. **Seizure in a Patient with a VP shunt** - Often due to CNS Infection or Malfunction of the Shunt. Consult a Neurosurgeon. Get CBC, CMP, Shunt series, CT Head. Neurosurgeon can Tap the Shunt for CSF if Infection is a concern.

3. **Neonatal:** A Neonate needs a Full Septic Workup and Admission in the event of a Seizure

4. **Status Epilepticus:** A Seizure that lasts at least 5 minutes without return to baseline. Need IV X 2, O2, Monitor. Assess Airway (Airway intervention is recommended in Status Epilepticus). Fingerstick Glucose. Labs (CBC, CMP, Lactate, UA, Urine Culture, Blood Culture, Toxicologic studies, HCG (Pregnancy test), Anticonvulsant levels, etc.), Note: During Status Epilepticus, First Control the Seizures! Best Management: Lorazepam. CT Head. LP if CNS infection is a possibility and No Contraindications (Don't do LP while patient is still seizing however).

SPINAL CORD COMPRESSION

1. **Spinal Cord Compression** - Emergent condition. May present with Back Pain, Leg Pain, Weakness/Motor Deficits, Sensory Deficits, Urinary Retention/Incontinence, Fecal Retention/Incontinence. Any of these are possible. Diagnosis is a Stat MRI. Stat Neurosurgery Consult (Radiation, Spine Surgery). Corticosteroids to Lessen Edema. Antibiotics if Epidural Abscess is Suspected. Note: Can occur in those with Malignancy, Epidural Abscess, etc.

STROKE

1. **Hemorrhagic**

   A) **Intracerebral:** Bleed in the Brain. Headache, Nausea, Vomiting. Risk Factors: tpA Administration for CVA, Use of Anticoagulants (ie. Warfarin), HTN, Trauma, Smoker, Cocaine use, AVM. Diagnosis: CT Head Noncontrast. Management: Airway, Neurosurgery Consult. Reverse Coagulopathy (ie FFP's, Vitamin K for Warfarin reversal). BP control but **Don't** allow Hypotension. Raise the Head of the bed. Stat Neurosurgery Consult. ICU Admit.

   B) **Subarachnoid:** Blood in the Subarachnoid Space. Severe Headache, Nausea, Vomiting, Neck Stiffness, Photophobia. Often due to Rupture of Aneurysm. Risks include HTN, Smoking, PCKD, Connective Tissue Disorders, Family History. Diagnosis: Noncontrast CT Head. If Head CT is Negative, Do LP (If No Contraindications). Positive finding is Xanthochromia (turns yellow on centrifuge) or Elevated RBC's (Note: Positive RBC's can also be due to a Traumatic Tap but if RBC's are still present in tubes 3, 4 consider it an SAH). SAH needs BP control so the patient doesn't rebleed but also **Avoid** hypotension. If Not contraindicated, give Nimodipine, to Prevent Vasospasm. Consult Neurosurgery Stat! ICU Admit.

2. Ischemic

A) Blood flow to the Brain is Blocked. Presents with Signs of Stroke: Weakness, Dizziness, Facial Droop, Dysarthria, Aphasia, Visual Changes, Sensory Changes, Ataxia, Headache, Confusion, etc.

B) **Embolic:** Sudden Onset generally. Usually due to Emboli, Myxoma, Vegetations on Valves

C) **Thrombotic:** Usually Gradual. Due to Hypercoagulability, Dissection, Atherosclerosis, etc.

D) **Diagnosis:** CT Head to r/o Hemorrhage and Possibly see Mild Ischemia, if possible. Stat Neurology Consult. Admit. If No hemorrhage and No contraindications, give Aspirin. If Persistent/Worsening Symptoms, if within the time frame of 3 hours (In some patients, within 4.5 hours), if risk of long term disability and fits all the inclusion criteria and if No contraindications, consider tPA (with Neurologist). On Admission, MRI, Echo, Carotid Doppler Ultrasound.

TRANSIENT CEREBRAL ISCHEMIA

Transient Ischemic Attack (TIA): Transient Neurological Symptom. Often under two hours. Very high risk of subsequent stroke. Do CT Head. If Negative for Bleed and No Contraindications, give Aspirin. Consult Neurology. These patients need to be Admitted for MRI, Echo, Carotid Doppler Ultrasound.

OBSTETRICS AND GYNECOLOGY

INFECTIOUS DISORDERS OF THE FEMALE GENITAL TRACT

1. Pelvic Inflammatory Disease (PID): Often due to Neisseria Gonorrhea and/or Chlamydia Trachomatis. Always treat both (also treat potential Trichomonas Vaginalis). PID often occurs in young patients with multiple sexual partners. Abdominal Pain. Vaginal Discharge. Fever. Pelvic Pain. Adnexal Tenderness. Cervical Motion Tenderness (CMT). Treatment: Antibiotics (ie Ceftriaxone + Azithromycin or Doxycycline + Flagyl is one option). The following patients need Admission: Pregnancy, Intractable Vomiting or Pain, High Fever, Very Abnormal Labs (ie. Very High WBC count or any other concerning findings), Toxic appearing, Septic, Comorbidities/Immunocompromised, Unreliable/Unable to follow up, Failed Outpatient Treatment, More Concerning Etiologies Cannot be Excluded, Concerning findings on Ultrasound that are worthy of Admission (ie. TOA, a Tubo-Ovarian Abscess). If a TOA is present, it warrants Admission. Concerning Complications of a PID include Ectopic Pregnancy and TOA.

2. Fitz Hugh-Curtis syndrome: Complication of PID (the infection ascends to the Liver). Leads to RUQ pain, Abdominal Pain and can present with PID symptoms. Diagnosis: Clinical, Ultrasound, CT Abdomen/Pelvis, Cultures. "Violin String Adhesions" can be found if a Laparotomy is conducted, in the Hepatic region. Treatment is Antibiotics (same ones used in PID). Admit.

3. Tuboovarian Abscess (TOA): Can be a Complication of PID often times but can also be secondary to other etiologies (ie. Complication of a disorder in the abdomen or even a complication of a Pelvic Surgical Procedure. The Physical Exam often demonstrates Unilateral Tenderness (CMT or Adnexal Tenderness). Abdominal Pain. Fever, Vaginal Discharge. Ultrasound is the Diagnosis. Treatment: IV Antibiotics and Admit to OBGYN for Possible Drainage in the OR.

OVARIES

1. Ovarian Torsion: The Ovary twists on its stalk. Risk of this occurring is a Lack of Blood Flow to the Ovary. Consider this in any woman with Abdominal Pain and/or Nausea/Vomiting, Pelvic Pain. Diagnosis: Ultrasound Transvaginal with Doppler (May show lack of blood flow to the ovary). Management: Stat OBGYN Consult and to the Operating Room for Lap. Keep in mind that a Patient can have Torsion and Detorsion so if it is High on your list of Suspicion, even with a Negative Ultrasound, Always Consult OBGYN. Note: Women with Ovarian Torsion can Torse and Detorse, so Always Consult OBGYN for any suspicion of Ovarian Torsion

VAGINA AND VULVA

1. **Bartholin's Abscess:** Abscess or Cyst on Duct of the Bartholin's Gland. Painful. Palpable Swelling/Mass. Management is a Word Catheter to Drain the Abscess

2. **Foreign Body:** Causes Discharge from the Vaginal Region. Do a Pelvic Exam and Remove it

3. **Vaginitis/Vulvovaginitis**

  a) **Bacterial Vaginosis:** Clue Cells on Microscopy. Patient with Vaginal Discharge with a "Fishy" Odor that is White/Grayish in Color. Treatment is Metronidazole.

  b) **Candidiasis:** Itchy, Red Vulva/Vagina. "Cottage Cheese, Curd-like" Discharge. Diagnosis is KOH for Pseudohyphae. Treatment is Fluconazole PO or Clotrimazole Cream

  c) **Trichomoniasis:** Vaginal Discharge. Occasionally Green. Diagnosis: Wet Prep shows Flagellated Trichomonads in Shapes of Pears. Treatment is Metronidazole

COMPLICATIONS OF PREGNANCY

1. **Abortion**

Note: Any Unstable Patient Needs Two Large Bore IV lines, O2, Monitor, Preop Labs, US (Bedside FAST), Stat OBGYN and OR.

The following applies to Stable Patients:
 - Pregnant patients need CBC, CMP, PT/PTT, Type and screen, Rh factor, B-HCG Quantitative, Urinalysis and an Ultrasound
 - If Rh Negative, give Rhogam
 - In a Pregnant Patient, prior to 20 weeks, get a Transvaginal Ultrasound. If BHCG is >1500 you should be able to see a viable pregnancy. If the BHCG is >1500 and No sign of a viable pregnancy is visible, keep Ectopic Pregnancy and Abortion on the Differential. If the BHCG is <1500, the diagnosis can still be the former, but it can also be too early in the pregnancy to visualize a viable pregnancy.

 - **Threatened:** Vaginal Bleeding, Closed Cervical Os, No Products of Conception. Needs Follow Up with OBGYN in 2 days for a Repeat US and BHCG, with Strict Follow Up and Return Instructions.

 - **Missed:** Prior to 20 weeks death of fetus. Needs D&C by OBGYN.

- **Incomplete:** Cervical Os is Open and there are Products of Conception Present on the Physical Exam. Some of the Conceptus is Passed. Products of Conception Present. Needs D&C by OBGYN.

- **Inevitable:** Vaginal Bleeding and a Cervical Os is Open. No Products of Conception. Needs D&C by OBGYN.

- **Complete:** All Fetal Tissue is passed with this Abortion that is Prior to 20 weeks Cervical os closed and Products of Conception Already Passed. Needs OBGYN Follow Up with Strict Follow Up and Return Instructions.

- **Septic:** Infection with Abortion. Fever, Pain, Foul Discharge, Tenderness on Pelvic Exam. Needs OBGYN Consult, IV Antibiotics and Admission.

2. **Ectopic Pregnancy:** A Pregnancy that is located outside the uterus (ie. Fallopian Tubes). Many Risk Factors exist (ie. Prior Ectopic Pregnancy, History of PID, etc.) but the majority of cases occur in those without any risk factors, so always keep this in the differential.
Signs/Symptoms: Vaginal Bleeding/Spotting and/or Abdominal Pain. Pelvic Exam may have CMT or Adnexal Tenderness. May have a Mass. May be Normal.
Send: CBC, CMP, PT/PTT, Type and Cross, Rh factor, B-HCG Quantitative, Urinalysis and an Ultrasound.
Diagnosis: Ultrasound and BHCG quantitative leads to the diagnosis. A Transvaginal Ultrasound should show a Viable Pregnancy or an Ectopic Pregnancy if the BHCG is > 1500.
Note: If the Patient is Unstable, be concerned about a Ruptured Ectopic Pregnancy. Give IVF's, PRBC's if Hypotensive shock from Blood loss, Get a Stat OBGYN Consult An Unstable Patient (Ruptured Ectopic Pregnancy) needs Immediate Surgical Intervention (to go to the OR with OBGYN for a Lap). An Unstable Ectopic Pregnancy can present with Hypotension from Blood Loss, Very Painful/Tender Abdomen, Peritoneal Signs.
A Stable patient should also have a Stat OBGYN Consult as well. A Stable patient can have Methotrexate as long as No Contraindications exist and the patient meets all the criteria for Medical Treatment as opposed to Surgical Treatment. It is given by the OBGYN. Note that Methotrexate **cannot** be given if there is Bleeding/a Ruptured Ectopic Pregnancy. It cannot be given if the patient is Unstable. It cannot be given if there is a Large sized Ectopic. It cannot be given if the patient has Failed Outpatient Management already. It cannot be given if the Patients Symptoms are worsening (i.e. Increasing Abdominal Pain). These cases all need Surgical intervention by the OBGYN. The Patient should be Admitted under the OBGYN.

3. **Heterotopic Pregnancy:** This is the presence of both an Intrauterine Pregnancy and an Ectopic Pregnancy. Note that those with Fertility Treatments are at Increased

Risk of Heterotopic Pregnancy. Needs OBGYN Consult for Surgical Intervention

4. **Molar Pregnancy** - Vaginal Bleeding. Grape like clusters on GU Exam. Ultrasound (US) shows a Snowstorm Pattern. Very Elevated BHCG Levels for Dates. Management: Stat OBGYN Consult for Intervention (ie. D&C)

5. **Preeclampsia:** In a Pregnant woman who is > 20 weeks old and can occur up to 6 weeks Postpartum. Manifests with Hypertension, Proteinuria, Edema, Visual changes, Headache. Always be cognizant that this can lead to Eclampsia (Seizure + Preeclampsia) so Prophylaxis with Magnesium is needed and Admission. For BP control, may try Hydrazine or Labetalol. Of Note: When giving Magnesium, Monitor the Deep Tendon Reflexes. If it is Decreased, then this could be Magnesium Toxicity, which can also lead to a Depression in the Respiratory Drive.

6. **Eclampsia:** A Pregnant patient with a Seizure and Preeclampsia. May have a Headache, Visual Changes and Other Symptoms listed above. Treatment is Magnesium and Delivery of the Baby. For BP Control can use Hydrazine or Labetalol

7. **Hemolysis, Elevated Liver enzymes, Low Platelets (HELLP) Syndrome** goes hand in hand with Preeclampsia/Eclampsia as it is a Severe form of Preeclampsia

8. **Gestational Trophoblastic Disease:** Excessive Growth of Trophoblastic Cells. Hydatidiform Mole (Partial or Complete), Choriocarcinoma. Nausea, Vomiting, Vaginal Bleeding, Vaginal exam may show Grape like Villi. Ultrasound with "Snowstorm" pattern. Very High BHCG levels (often >100,000) and often an Enlarged Uterus. Tx: OBGYN Consult and Admit in order to Evacuate the Uterus and Send the Tissue for Sampling. Choriocarcinoma needs Chemotherapy

9. **Abruptio Placentae:** Placenta separates from Uterus. Abdominal Pain, Possible Vaginal Bleeding. Increased Risk in patients with prior episodes or Cocaine users/ Smokers/Preeclampsia/Trauma/HTN. Clinical Diagnosis. **Don't** do a Pelvic exam until you know it is **NOT** Placental Previa because this can lead to Massive Bleeding! Monitor the Fetus. Get a Stat OBGYN Consult. Treatment is Emergent Delivery (C-Section)

10. **Placenta Previa:** Part of Placenta is over the Cervix. Causes Painless Bleeding during/after the Second Trimester. **Contraindications** in Placenta Previa or Suspicion of it is a Pelvic exam (Never do a Pelvic Exam in Placenta Previa as it can lead to a Massive Hemorrhage!)

11. **Hyperemesis Gravidarum:** Excessive Nausea, Vomiting. Labs: Low Potassium Possible and Ketonemia. Dehydration. Tx: IV Hydration with 5% Dextrose in NS, an Antiemetic. Admit if No resolution of Ketonemia/Electrolyte Imbalances/Symptoms

COMPLICATIONS OF LABOR

1. **Premature Labor:** Labor before 37 weeks. Contractions. OBGYN needed. Admit. Possible Tocolytics, Steroids.

2. **Premature Rupture Of Membranes:** Membranes Rupture before Labor. Nitrazine Paper Test Positive (Blue), Ferning. OBGYN for Admission

COMPLICATIONS OF DELIVERY

1. **Nuchal Cord:** Often times the Cord is around the Neck. Needs to be Delivered Immediately

2. **Prolapse of Cord:** Cord is on the verge of coming out before the rest of the baby. Management: Manually hold cord up until patient reaches the OR for Emergency C-section

3. **Breech Delivery:** The Rear End is at the Opening During Delivery. Best Management is C-section.

4. **Shoulder Dystocia:** Shoulder is difficult to deliver during the delivery of the baby. May attempt Mc Roberts Maneuver in which the mother places flexed legs in a Knee to Chest Position Alignment. May also consider an Episiotomy as an adjunct.

POSTPARTUM COMPLICATIONS

1. **Endometritis:** Abdominal pain, Fever, Foul Smelling Discharge, CMT, Tender Uterus. Needs IV Antibiotics

2. **Hemorrhage:** Needs Labs (CBC, CMP, PT/PTT, Type and Cross, IVF's, PRBC's). Differential: Uterine Atony (Treatment is Uterine Massage and Oxytocin), Uterine Rupture (Treatment is IVF's, IV Antibiotics, Type and Cross for Possible PRBC Transfusion, Laparotomy Stat with Stat OBGYN), Retained Placenta, Inverted Uterus, Laceration, Bleeding Disorder

3. **Mastitis:** Red, Swollen, Tender Breast. Needs Antibiotics and Warm Compresses

4. **Uterine Rupture:** Abdominal Pain, Vaginal Bleeding. More often in those with a History of C-sections. Management: IVF's, Possible PRBC's, IV Antibiotics, Needs Stat OR with OBGYN for Stat C-section

RENAL AND UROGENITAL

1. **Acute Renal Failure:**

    1. **Pre-Renal** is often due to Volume Depletion. The Management is Replete Volume and Manage Underlying Cause.

    2. **Intrinsic** is due to a Structural abnormality, a Toxin or a Medication or Ischemia. Management is to Discontinue the Causative Toxin/Medication, to Treat the Underlying Infection, to Treat the Underlying Cause.

    3. **Post-Renal** is due to an Obstruction (ie. BPH, Tumor, etc). The Management is to Manage the Underlying Obstruction (ie. Foley).

2a. **Complications of Renal Dialysis:** Electrolyte abnormalities, Thrombosis, Bleeding, Infections, Hypotension, Dysrhythmias

2b. **Indications for Dialysis:** Electrolyte disorders (ie. Hyperkalemia), Acidosis, Edema, Ingestion of Toxic substances (ie. Salicylates, Methanol, Ethylene Glycol), Uremia

3. **Glomerular Disorders**

A. **Glomerulonephritis:** Inflamed Glomerulus. Can be due to Streptococcal Infection (Poststreptococcal Glomerulonephritis = PSGN) or due to certain systemic diseases, such as Lupus. PSGN presents with Hematuria, HTN, Edema. Needs Antibiotics if due to PSGN.

B. **Nephrotic syndrome:** Proteinuria, Edema, Hyperlipidemia. These Patients are at Increased risk for Blood Clots

4. **Infection**

A. **Cystitis:** Urinary tract infection. Symptoms of Dysuria, Increased Urinary Frequency. May have a Positive Urinalysis. Send Urine Culture. Treat with Antibiotics.

B. **Pyelonephritis:** Infection of Kidney. Often secondary to a UTI that ascends from Bladder to the Kidney. Positive CVA tenderness. Needs IV Antibiotics and Admission.

5. Male Genital Tract Disorders

A. Balanitis: Inflamed Glans Penis. These Need Appropriate Hygiene. Can use Antibiotics. If due to Candida, use an Antifungal agent. Steroid Cream

B. Balanoposthitis: Inflamed Glans and Penile Foreskin (Prepuce). These Need Appropriate Hygiene. Can use Antibiotics. If due to Candida, use an Antifungal agent. Steroid Cream.

C. Epididymitis: Inflammation of the Epididymis. Testicular Pain. Possible Positive Urinalysis. Needs Ultrasound (US) of the Testicles with Doppler flow to rule out Testicular Torsion. Management of Epididymitis is Antibiotics (In young men, cover with Gonorrhea and Chlamydia Coverage Antibiotics, including Ceftriaxone and Doxycycline. In Older men, cover for other organisms with Ciprofloxacin).

D. Gangrene of the Scrotum (Fournier's Gangrene): Painful, Tender, Swollen Scrotal area. May See Bullae. Discoloration. Crepitus. Fournier's Gangrene is essentially a Necrotizing Fasciitis of the Perineum. Needs Stat Surgery Consult for Surgical Debridement and IV Antibiotics

E. Prostatitis: Inflammation/Infection of the Prostate. Increased Urinary Frequency Possible. Dysuria possible. Fever possible. Rectal exam with a Tender Prostate. Send Cultures. Needs Antibiotics x 4 weeks and Urology Follow Up. (In young men under age 35, cover with Gonorrhea and Chlamydia Coverage Antibiotics, including Ceftriaxone and Doxycycline. In Older men, cover for other organisms with Ciprofloxacin). Provide Specialty Follow-Up. If patient is ill-appearing, Admit.

F. Urethritis: In younger populations, consider Gonococcal Urethritis. They may have Dysuria or be Asymptomatic. Needs Ceftriaxone, Azithromycin. Send culture samples from the GU region. Treat the Partner(s).

G. Paraphimosis: Penis Foreskin is Retracted and Nonreducible. It can cut off blood supply without prompt management. May attempt Manual Reduction (ie. Place slight pressure on glans penis for a few minutes intermittently) and if this does not work, Stat Urology Consult. Possible Dorsal Slit. This is Emergent.

H. Phimosis: Penis Foreskin is Reduced and Cannot be Retracted. Needs Urologist to follow up for Possible Circumcision

I. Priapism: Erection that is Painful and Unanticipated. May occur in Sickle Cell Anemia, Drug use, Patients with Malignancy, etc. For Sickle Cell Anemia Patients, Management: IV Hydration, Oxygen, Pain Medications, Exchange Transfusion. For others with Priapism, a Stat Urology Consultation for Phenylephrine Injection via

Corporal Aspiration/Irrigation and Possible OR. Needs Admission.

J. **Testicular Torsion:** Torsing of the Testicle leading to cut off of Blood Flow. Abdominal Pain, Testicular Pain, Nausea, Vomiting. On Physical Examination: Possible Absent Cremasteric Reflex. Possible Abnormal Horizontal Testicular Lie. Tender, Swollen Testicle. Stat Urology Consult. Diagnosis: Ultrasound of Testicles with Doppler Flow would show lack of blood flow. If US is normal and there is still clinical suspicion, Stat Urology Consult and Admit. In the interim, Manual Reduction could be attempted in those with Definite Torsion. Stat Urology Consult for OR for Surgical Repair for Torsion.

NEPHRITIS

1. **Hemolytic Uremic Syndrome:** ART (Anemia, Renal failure, Thrombocytopenia) - See Oral Boards Section

STRUCTURAL DISORDERS

1. **Calculus of Urinary Tract:** Kidney Stone or Stone in the Urinary Tract (ie Ureter). Diagnosis: CT Abdomen/Pelvis Noncontrast. Treatment is IV Hydration, attempt to Collect the stone in a Strainer and Urology Follow Up. Indications for Admission are Concomitant Infection, Obstruction, Stone > 5 mm, Nausea/Vomiting, Intractable, Persistent Uncontrolled Pain, Unreliable Follow Up, Comorbidities, Pregnancy, Immunocompromised, Elderly.

2. **Uremic Encephalopathy:** AMS, Weakness. Can lead to Bleeding. Can lead to Effusion. Needs Hemodialysis.

INDICATIONS FOR EMERGENT HEMODIALYSIS

Indications for Emergent Hemodialysis: Acidosis, Uremia, Fluid Overload, Hyperkalemia, Toxins/Ingestions (ie. Ethylene Glycol, Salicylate).

PULMONARY

ACUTE UPPER AIRWAY DISORDERS

1. **Croup:** Laryngotracheitis. "Barking Cough". URI symptoms, Fever, Hoarse voice, Worse at Night, Worse in the Winter and Early Spring, Often due to Parainfluenza. Severe = Shortness of Breath, Stridor. X-ray shows Steeple sign. Often in kids age 6 months to 5 years. Needs Oxygen, Cool Mist, Racemic Epinephrine Nebulizers, Dexamethasone, Fluids.

2. **Epiglottitis:** Infection of the Epiglottis. Patient often is in Respiratory Distress, Tripod position, is more comfortable Sitting Forward. Drooling, High Fever, Stridor, Sore Throat, Odynophagia. Keep the patient Comfortable. Keep parents in the room with the child. Occurs in Children and in Unimmunized Adults. Give Oxygen. May Confirm with Bedside Lateral Neck Soft Tissue X-ray if needed (Shows Thumbprint Sign which is the Enlarged Swollen Epiglottis). Consult Anesthesiology, ENT, Surgery, ICU/PICU and Admit. Patient needs to go to OR. Airway is the # 1 priority with the most skilled staff. IV Antibiotics. Some also give IV Steroids.

OBSTRUCTIVE

1. **Foreign body in Airway:** Coughing, Gagging. Wheezing. X-ray. Needs Bronchoscopy in OR. Consult ENT, Pulmonary.

2. **Bronchiolitis:** Usually due to RSV. Hx of URI. Wheezing in an infant, often in the winter months. Retractions, Increased RR. CXR. May try Albuterol, Racemic Epinephrine. Can give Dexamethasone. Admit if Retractions/Labored Breathing, Toxic, Comorbidity, Hypoxic, No improvement after Observation or Premature or Under 6 months old, Unreliable Follow Up, Concomitant Infection.

3. **Asthma:** This is an Inflammatory Disease. Often causes Wheezing. In severe cases, the patient may be fatigued, in respiratory distress and not moving air. Management: Albuterol, Atrovent, Steroids (Prednisone or Solumedrol), Oxygen. If Not working, Consider Magnesium, Epinephrine.

4. **COPD (Chronic Obstructive pulmonary Disease):** Shortness of Breath, Wheezing. May have a Productive Cough. Tx: Oxygen, Albuterol/Atrovent, Steroids (Methylprednisolone), Antibiotics (to cover concomitant pneumonia). If no improvement, consider Bipap

5. **Cystic Fibrosis:** Thick Secretions cause Pulmonary Issues (Thick Secretions, Productive Cough), Infections, GI Issues (SBO, etc). Treatment is Antibiotics, Oxygen, Chest Physiotherapy. Consult Pulmonary.

PLEURAL DISORDERS, MEDIASTINAL DISORDERS, CHEST WALL DISORDERS

1. **Pleural Effusion:** Fluid accumulation in the Lungs. Chest pain, Cough, Dyspnea. Can be due to Cancer, Trauma, Comorbidities (ie. SLE), CHF, etc. CXR shows Blunted Costophrenic Angle. Thoracentesis to see the content of the Pleural fluid. Transudates (CHF, Nephrotic syndrome, etc.) Exudate (Infection, Cancer, etc).

2. **Pneumomediastinum:** Chest Pain, Hamman's Crunch (when auscultating the heart), Trouble Swallowing, Crepitus, Subcutaneous Emphysema. Admit to ensure that there are no Concerning Etiologies for the Pneumomediastinum.

3. **Pneumothorax:** Collapsed Lung. Presents with Possible Chest Pain and Dyspnea.

    A) **Simple** - Unilateral Absent breath sounds. CXR shows Pneumothorax (Absence of lung markings to the edge of the field). Physical Exam: Hyperresonance and Absent lung sounds on the side of the Pneumothorax. Management is Chest tube

    B) **Tension** - JVD, Unilateral Absent Breath sounds, Tracheal Deviation. Dx is Clinical. Treatment is Needle Decompression and then a Chest Tube

4. **Empyema** - Pus in Pleural Region. Presents with Dyspnea, Fever. Can be secondary to infection (ie Pneumonia, Abscess), Trauma, etc.

5. **Mediastinitis:** Chest Pain, Dyspnea, Fever. May Feel Crepitus, Subcutaneous Emphysema. CXR, CT scan. Management: IV Antibiotics, Cardiothoracic Surgery Consultation. An Etiology for this that is very Concerning is Boerhaave's Syndrome.

PULMONARY EMBOLISM

1. **Venous thromboembolism:** Pulmonary embolism is a Blood Clot in the Pulmonary Vasculature

    a. **Pulmonary Embolism:** Blood Clot in the Lung Vasculature. Chest Pain, Dyspnea, Possible Hemoptysis. May have had Recent Leg Pain or Swelling. Possible Back pain, Syncope, New Wheezing. Tachycardia, Tachypnea.

PE Risk factors: History of PE or DVT, History of Familial blood disorders (Thrombophilias) that Predispose to Clotting, Prolonged Immobilization (Long Travel, Surgery recently in the past one month or so, Bed bound, Obesity), Oral Contraceptive Use, Pregnancy, Old age, Trauma, Malignancy, CHF

Wells Criteria: Scoring system to ascertain the likelihood of a PE: DVT symptoms (3), Diagnosis of PE is most likely than another diagnosis (1), Prior DVT or PE (1.5), HR >100 (1.5), Surgery/immobilization (1.5), Malignancy (1), Hemoptysis (1); A score > 4 is more likely a PE. (As an alternate method: <2 Low Risk, 2-6 Moderate Risk, >6 High Risk).

Diagnosis: CTA Chest unless Contraindications exist. Use V/Q scan if Renal Failure present. Reminder: D-dimer is only used to try to rule out PE in LOW risk patients. It does not work for moderate or high risk patients. EKG could be normal or may have sinus tachycardia. It could also show some Right ventricular strain. It could also show S1Q3T3. CXR can be normal or may show Hampton's hump or Westermark's sign.

Treatment: Heparin or LMWH (Contraindicated in Renal Failure Patients). These can be bridged with Coumadin later. If Anticoagulation is contraindicated, IVC filter may be placed temporarily. Do not use LMWH on patients with renal disease because it is renally cleared and if renally impaired patient, it won't clear and can lead to bleeding. Can give Heparin and later bridge with Coudamin. If the patient has a Massive PE and is Hemodynamically Unstable (ie Hypotensive, Hypoxic, etc.), use Thrombolytics. For Hypotension, can consider Vasopressors (Dobutamine). Intubation and ICU Admission. Disposition: Admit

Types of Embolism: Thrombus (Blood clot), Amniotic Fluid (Pregnant patient), Fat (Fat Embolism, often after Long Bone Fractures presents with Dyspnea, Petechiae, Altered Mental Status), Air (Air Embolism). DVT is a Blood Clot in the Deep Veins of the Legs. Pulmonary Embolism: Blood clot in the Lung Vasculature.

PULMONARY INFECTIONS

1. **Lung Abscess:** Abscess in the Lung. Chest Pain, Dyspnea, Cough, Fever. Diagnosis is an imaging study (ie CT Scan). Treatment is IV Antibiotics, for instance, Clindamycin.

2. **Pneumonia:**
Productive Cough, Fever, Weakness. PORT score, CURB-65 score
Aspiration Pneumonia: A Pneumonia that often occurs in a patient who vomits/ regurgitates (ie alcoholics) due to anaerobes
Community-acquired: in those who have not recently been hospitalized. Does not use health care facilities often. Generally the treatment entails: Azithromycin + Ceftriaxone
Health care-associated: Pneumonia that begins more than 2 days after entering the

hospital. Anyone Hospitalized within past 90 days. Anyone who lives in a Nursing home or was Recently Hospitalized (within the past 4 weeks), Dialysis patients, or Anyone who uses Healthcare facilities often. The Antibiotics required for this are more Broad Spectrum Coverage

3. **Pulmonary Tuberculosis:** A bacterium that often occurs in endemic areas, incarcerated patients, immunosuppressed patients, etc. It causes Night Sweats, Weight Loss, Hemoptysis, etc. Need isolation. Send sputum AFB samples. Needs treatment with the regimen (e. Rifampin, Ethambutol, Pyrazinamide, INH).

4. **Pertussis:** Whooping cough. Three phases exist (Catarrhal Phase: URI for a week or two, Paroxysmal Phase: Whooping Cough for 2 to 4 weeks, Convalescent Phase: Continue to Cough for Weeks). Whooping cough for over two weeks. Supportive Treatment. Antibiotic may shorten the course.

NONCARDIOGENIC PULMONARY EDEMA

1. Causes of this are Medications/Drugs (ie. Salicylates, Opiates, etc.), HAPE (Best Management is Descent!), ARDS, Aspiration, Sepsis, Head Trauma, etc.

TRACHEOSTOMY TUBE COMPLICATIONS

1. Infection
2. Esophageal Injury
3. Dislodgment
4. Trauma to Nerves, Vessels
5. Respiratory Distress
6. Hemorrhage
7. Pneumothorax
8. Air Embolism
9. Pneumomediastinum
10. Subcutaneous Emphysema

SEPTIC EMBOLI

1. An Infected Embolus that travels to other parts of the body
2. Often caused by Endocarditis
3. May present with Malaise, Murmur, Rash, Pain and a Fever (Also Possible depending on the site: Headache, Seizure, etc.)
4. Needs Blood Cultures and an Echocardiogram (CT scan, etc.)
5. Management is IV Antibiotics

TOXICOLOGY

In the Toxicologic Patient, Check a FSG and be certain to send all of the Labs (CBC, CMP, PT/PTT, Acetaminophen level, Salicylate level, Alcohol Level, UA, UTox, EKG, HCG, ABG, etc...ie. Digoxin level, Iron level etc. depending on the case scenario). Consult Poison Control. Manage with Antidote, Supportive Measures and Disposition Accordingly (will usually Entail Observation for at least a few hours or more likely, Admission).

1. **Acetaminophen:** May be Asymptomatic. May be Symptomatic. Nausea, Vomiting, Weakness, Abdominal pain. Abnormal labs, Lactic acidosis, Elevated LFTs, Elevated Acetaminophen Level. Coagulopathy, Renal Failure. Check Acetaminophen Level at Present and also at 4 hours Post Ingestion. Check FSG. Also send CBC, CMP, PT/PTT, Toxicologic Levels: Acetaminophen level, Salicylate level, Alcohol Level, Urinalysis, Urine Toxicologic Screen, EKG, HCG, Consult Poison Control). Acetaminophen Level: Plot on the Rumack-Matthew Nomogram. Give NAC. NAC is the most beneficial in the first 8 hours after ingestion. Always strongly consider giving NAC in Tylenol Overdose Scenarios. Admit.

2. **Nonsteroidal Anti-Inflammatories (NSAIDS):** GI Bleeding, Renal Failure, AMS, Vomiting, Abdominal Pain. Check FSG. Send all Labs (CBC, CMP, PT/PTT and Toxicologic Levels: Acetaminophen level, Salicylate level, Alcohol Level, UA, UTox, EKG, HCG). If Minimal to No symptoms, Observe for at least 6 hours. If co-ingestion of other substances or more severe symptoms, Admit. If AMS or Seizure, Manage Airway. If Seizure, Give Benzodiazepine. If any Concerning symptoms (Dysrhythmia, Hypotension, AMS, Seizure, Renal Failure, GI Bleed, etc, Admit!)

3. **Salicylates:** Respiratory Alkalosis and Metabolic Acidosis, Tinnitus, Nausea, Vomiting, Dizziness, Hearing Loss, Fever, Diaphoresis, Ataxia, Increased Respiratory Rate, Increased Heart Rate, Shock, Dysrhythmias, Pulmonary issues, Altered Mental Status, Seizure, Renal Failure, Pulmonary Edema. Diagnosis is Salicylate level. Send all the labs listed above as well, in addition to an ABG. Management is IV, O2, Monitor. Normal saline, Sodium Bicarbonate, Consider Hemodialysis (if level >100 in Acute ingestion or >60 in a Chronic ingestion, AMS, Neurological symptoms, Renal failure, Bleeding, Pulmonary involvement, Renal Involvement, etc). ICU Admission.

4. **Ethylene Glycol:** Renal failure, Altered Mental Status, Acidosis, CHF, Respiratory issues. Management is Fomepizole

5. **Methanol:** Visual changes (Blurry), Altered Mental Status, Nausea/Vomiting. Anion Gap Acidosis. Management is Fomepizole

6. **Anticholinergics:** Altered Mental Status, Red skin, Dry skin, Urinary Retention, Hyperthermia, Mydriasis, Constipation. Dysrhythmia, Possible Seizure (use standard seizure treatment). Management is Supportive and Treat Symptoms with Standard treatments. Admit to Observation

Mnemonic: MY DREAMS (**MY**driasis, **D**ysrhythmias, **D**ry Skin, **R**etention (Constipation, Urinary Retention), **E**rythema (Red Skin), **AMS, S**eizure (and Hyperthermia) = **Anticholinergic Mnemonic**

7. **Cholinergics:** ie. Organophosphates, Carbamates (Insecticides): Lacrimation, Rhinorrhea, Salivation, Diarrhea, Nausea, Vomiting, Weakness, Urination. Treatment: Manage Airway, Atropine, Pralidoxime (2-PAM). Admit to ICU

8. **Anticoagulants:** Heparin, Warfarin. Can lead to Bleeding. Should send PT/PTT in addition to the usual labs and Manage accordingly. ie. Heparin Reversal is with Protamine. Warfarin Reversal is with Vitamin K, FFP, depending on active bleeding, etc.

9. **TCAs (Tricyclic Antidepressants):** For instance: Amitriptyline. Altered Mental Status, Seizure, Dysrhythmia, Tachycardia. EKG: Wide QRS, Positive R wave in aVR with a Terminal R wave, S in lead I is Negative). Hypotension needs IV fluids. Seizure needs Benzodiazepines. Any Cardiac issue (Prolonged QRS, Conduction issues, Dysrhythmias) Needs Sodium Bicarbonate. Note: Sodium Bicarbonate can cause Hypokalemia so measure Potassium frequently and do repeat EKG's. Treat Torsades with Magnesium, etc.

10. **Serotonin Syndrome:** Due to medications that increase serotonin. Altered Mental Status, Weakness, Fever, Confusion, Diarrhea, Tremor, Hyperreflexia, Trismus, Seizure, Rigidity, Myoclonus, Sweating, Abnormal Blood Pressure. Treatment is to Stop all serotonergic medications. Give Cyproheptadine. For Rigidity, Benzodiazepine can be given. ICU Admission.

11. **Neuroleptic Malignant Syndrome:** Fever, Rigidity, AMS, Hyperthermia. BP Variability. Tachycardia. Can cause Renal issues. Management: Stop the medication causing this. IV fluids. Cooling if Hyperthermic. Admit.

12. **Carbon Monoxide:** Headache, Seizure, Weakness, Confusion, Chest Pain, Dizziness, Dysrhythmias, Dyspnea, Ataxia, Nausea, Vomiting, Visual changes. Diagnosis: Carboxyhemoglobin level. Management: 100% Oxygen or HBO in some candidates (Pregnancy, MI, AMS, Syncope, Neurological symptoms/signs). Multiple family members, pets may all be symptomatic at the same time. More common in the winter due to space heaters, etc. Admit.

13. **Digitalis:** Inhibits Na-K ATPase pump —> Hyperkalemia and Hyponatremia. Nausea, Vomiting, Diarrhea, Dysrhythmias, Weakness, Confusion, Abdominal Pain, AMS. For Hyperkalemia Treatment: (Note: Calcium is **CONTRAINDICATED** in Patients on Digoxin!): Insulin, Glucose, Sodium Bicarbonate, Digoxin Specific Fab Antibody Fragments, Kayexalate, Hemodialysis. Hypomagnesemia: Replete as long as Renal Functioning is Normal. Cardiac Arrest: Follow ACLS but please give Digoxin specific Fab Antibody fragments as well! All Cardiac dysrhythmias: in addition to standard ACLS, give Digoxin specific Fab Antibody fragments as well!

14. **Beta Blockers:** Bradycardia, Hypotension, AV blocks, Dysrhythmia, Altered Mental Status, Seizure, Respiratory Distress. Can get Hypoglycemic. Send Labs, EKG. IVF's. If still Hypotensive, Vasopressors. Management: Glucagon. Admit.

15. **Calcium Channel Blockers:** Bradycardia, Hypotension, AV blocks, Altered Mental Status. Can get Hyperglycemic. Send Labs, EKG. IVF's. If still Hypotensive, Vasopressors. Management: Insulin. Dextrose. Admit.

16. **Cocaine:** Can lead to Intracranial Hemorrhage, Myocardial Infarction, Seizure, Pneumothorax, Rhabdomyolysis, Bowel Ischemia, Pregnancy Complications (ie. Abruptio Placentae). Diagnosis: Blood Toxicology Studies, Urine Toxicology Studies. Management is dependent on the Presentation. Benzodiazepines, etc. (See oral boards section)

17. **Cyanide:** Hypertension, Bradycardia, Tachycardia, Altered Mental Status, Headache, Seizure, Shortness of Breath. Causes Lactate Elevation and Metabolic Acidosis. Treatment: Oxygen, IVF's, Inhaled Amyl Nitrite, IV Sodium Nitrite, IV Sodium Thiosulfate. Another Management Regimen that can be used is IV Hydroxocobalamin.

18. **Hydrogen Sulfide:** Causes Nausea, Vomiting, Headache. Treatment: Decontaminate, Oxygen and then you can give IV Sodium Nitrite.

19. **Hypoglycemics/Insulin:** Cause Hypoglycemia. Sulfonylurea ingestion/overdose needs Admission and so does Moderate to Long acting Insulin (to ensure no Rebound Hypoglycemia, due to their longer half lives). Treatment is Dextrose. For Sulfonylurea ingestion, the Treatment is Dextrose and Octreotide.

20. **Iron:** Stage I - GI (Nausea, Vomiting, Diarrhea, Abdominal Pain), Stage II - Latent Phase is Asymptomatic (Note: Doesn't always occur), Stage III - Coagulopathy, Lactic Acidosis, Shock, Stage IV - Liver Toxicity. Diagnosis: Serum Iron Level, CBC, CMP, PT/PTT, ABG, X-ray Abdomen/KUB. Treatment: For those with symptoms, Whole Bowel Irrigation with PEG, Deferoxamine, IVF's.

21. **Marine Toxins:** Note that Jellyfish, which are Nematocysts cause a very painful lesion, Nausea, Vomiting. Can even cause Cardiac Arrest. With Jellyfish Stings, you need to place Vinegar on the Lesion. Give Pain Medications.
Note: Stingrays (Stingers) present with the same/similar symptoms but you need to place Hot Water on the Lesion.

22. **Methemoglobinemia:** Headache, Tachycardia, Weakness. Give Oxygen but you notice that it does not improve the symptoms. Tx: Methylene Blue, ICU admission

23. **Mushrooms:** The later the onset of Nausea/Vomiting/Symptoms, the worse it is. If Symptomatic, Admit for Observation.

24. **Organophosphates:** Salivation, Urinary incontinence, Vomiting, Abdominal pain, Diarrhea, Lacrimation, Bradycardia, Dyspnea. If intubation needed for airway protection, do **Not** use succinylcholine. Decontamination (remove clothing etc), Atropine, Pralidoxime. Admit.

25. **Opioids:** AMS, Miosis, Fatigue, Respiratory issues are all possible. Treatment is Naloxone (Narcan), Airway Management, Admit.

26. **Sympathomimetics (ie. Cocaine):** AMS, Tachycardia, Mydriasis. Treatment: Benzodiazepine, etc. Admit. (See Oral Boards section)

27. **Chemical Warfare Agents:** (Sarin, Ricin, etc.) - See the Section on Infectious disorders

28. **Scromboid Poisoning:** Due to Histamine. Fish poisoning. Causes Nausea, Vomiting, Diarrhea, Possible Rash, Abdominal Pain, Flushed skin, Swelling, Respiratory Distress. Treatment is Benadryl. If concerning symptoms, Admit.

29. **Hydrogen Fluoride:** Very painful when exposed to the skin. Fluoride binds Calcium and causes Hypocalcemia. It can also lead to much more dangerous scenarios like Dysrhythmias. Management is Irrigation and Calcium Repletion.

30. **Lithium:**
Acute: Nausea, Vomiting
Chronic: Weakness, AMS
Send all labs, Toxicologic levels and Lithium Level
Management: IVF's and Hemodialysis (For Neurological symptoms like Seizure, Confusion)

31. **Strychnine:** Severe Muscle Contractions, Opisthotonos. Management: Airway Management and Benzodiazepines for the Muscle Contractions

32. Arsenic:
Acute: Nausea, Vomiting, Diarrhea, Dysrhythmias, Renal Issues
Chronic: Neurological Findings (Paresthesias)
Management: Airway Management as Needed, Benzodiazepine for Seizure. Whole Bowel Irrigation with PEG (Polyethylene Glycol). For the Arsenic poisoned patients who are symptomatic, consider BAL (Dimercaprol) for Chelation. Admit.

33. Isopropanol: Nausea, Vomiting, GI Bleed, CNS Depression, AMS, Hypotensive, Respiratory Distress. Labs show: Ketonemia, Ketonuria, Elevated Osmolal Gap. No Acidosis. Check FSG, Send all labs (CBC, CMP, PT/PTT, Type & Screen, Acetaminophen Level, Salicylate Level, Alcohol Level, Isopropanolol Level, Acetone Level, etc). Management: IVF's, Consider Hemodialysis, Admit.

34. Ciguatera Poisoning: It causes Headache, Paresthesias around the Mouth, Vomiting, Abdominal Pain, Paresthesias when a Cold Sensation is felt, Bodyaches, Nausea, Vomiting, Diarrhea. Possible Bradycardia. Possible Hypotension. Management is IVF's and Symptomatic Treatment. IVF's. May consider Mannitol.

TRAUMA

A. General Trauma Management Guideline:

1. **Airway Management:** Can the Patient Speak? Is the Airway Compromised already or will it get compromised soon? Should you Prophylactically Intubate? Immobilize the C-Spine at this time as well

2. **Breathing:** Inspect the Chest. Wounds? Abnormal Movement? Tracheal Deviation? Auscultate Lungs: Breath Sounds Equal and Bilateral? Normal Breath Sounds? Palpate: Crepitus? Percuss.
For instance: A Tension Pneumothorax needs Stat Needle Decompression and then a Chest Tube. Is there an Open Pneumothorax? Needs a 3 sided Occlusive Dressing.

3. **Circulation:** Color (Pale? Gray?), Pulses, Capillary Refill, Look for JVD, Auscultate Heart Sounds. Look for Obvious Blood Loss and Control the Bleeding with Pressure. Give IVF's/PRBC's if Hypotensive Shock (ie. Hemorrhagic Shock). Cardiac Tamponade Management if Present: Pericardiocentesis.

4. **Disability:** (This is the Initial Neuro Examination: GCS Score) - Reminder that later you may need to consider a CT Head, CT C-Spine (Complete the Full Neurological Exam later)

5. **Exposure:** This is when you Expose the rest of the body in order to ensure that no life threatening injuries are being missed. Note: Remember to Cover the Body with a Blanket after examining each portion, in order to Prevent Hypothermia. You will Maintain In-line C-Spine Immobilization, while you and your colleagues temporarily Log-roll the patient onto his/her side in order to Inspect/Palpate the Back and Do a Rectal Exam. Note: Control Bleeding of an Unstable Pelvic Fracture with a Pelvic Binder (Will Need OR). An Ultrasound FAST should be done on the Abdomen to look for a Positive FAST Exam, which would need to go to the OR (Intraperitoneal Bleeding). In a Patient with an Extremity Fracture, do a Neurovasculature Check, Control any Bleeding with Pressure, and Consult Orthopedics. Also Note that a Modified FAST Exam can be used to look for a Pneumothorax and Cardiac Tamponade as well, so that you can implement Ultrasound at the beginning during the Breathing/Circulation section, in order to look for these. Note: Trauma Cases all Need a Stat Trauma Consult.

B. Abdominal Trauma

Unstable? —> IV X 2, Monitor, O2, Labs (CBC, Type and Cross, etc), IVF's, PRBC's possibly, Stat Surgery/Trauma Consult and OR!

1. **Penetrating** - For instance: Stab wound, GSW. A GSW needs to go STAT to the OR (Stat Surgery consult)

2. **Retroperitoneum** - ie. Duodenum, Kidneys, etc. A CT scan is more useful to find Retroperitoneal injuries and most injuries in this section

3. Note: **Only send Stable patients for CT scans!**

4. **Solid Organ** - ie. Liver, Spleen (CT scan with IV contrast visualizes the details the best if the patient is stable enough)

5. **US FAST** Study (See if Positive for Fluid) —> If Positive for Intraperitoneal Fluid, Patient Unstable —> Immediately to OR with Surgery for Laparotomy because indicative of Intra-Abdominal Hemorrhage

6. **Other Surgical Indications** (OR for Laparotomy) —> Unstable Patient (ie. Hypotensive), Positive FAST exam, Rebound/Guarding (Peritoneal), GSW, Diaphragm injured, Ruptured Viscous

7. **Liver Injury** —> Possible Hemorrhage. May be visualized on CT scan with IV contrast, if the patient is stable. Management is Surgical if Unstable. If patient is Stable and the CT results are minor, Admit for Observation (Repeat Labs, Monitoring, Repeat Abdominal Examinations, etc. and if these become concerning, then must go to OR). If the patient is Unstable or there are concerning findings on the CT (Moderate to Severe Hemorrhage, High Grade Injury), then patient needs to go to the OR. Management is Laparotomy if Unstable Patient or if there is a High Grade Injury.

8. **Splenic Injury** —> Possible Hemorrhage. May be visualized on CT scan with IV Contrast, if the Patient is Stable. Management is Surgical if Unstable. If the Patient is Stable and the CT results are minor, Admit for Observation (Repeat Labs, Monitoring, Repeat Abdominal Examinations and if these become concerning, then the patient must go to the OR). If the patient is Unstable or there are concerning findings on the CT (Moderate to Severe Hemorrhage), then the Patient needs to go to the OR.

9. **Diaphragmatic Injury:** Chest Pain, Shortness of Breath. Diagnosis: Chest X-ray. CT scan. If the studies are inconclusive and you have a High suspicion, send the patient to the OR (Laparotomy). Management is a Stat Surgical Consult for a Laparotomy to Repair it.

10. **Pancreas Injury:** Definitive Diagnosis and Management often entails Surgical Intervention, especially if it's a Higher stage injury

C. Chest Trauma

1. **Aortic Injury:** Can occur as a Deceleration injury. May have Back pain, Chest pain, and other symptoms. CXR may present with a Widened Mediastinum, Loss of Aortic Knob, Blurred Arch of the Aorta and Other findings. Diagnosis: CT Chest. Needs a Stat Surgery Consult for Immediate Operative Repair in the OR.

2. **Flail Chest:** Asymmetry in the Movement of the Chest Wall Cavity due to Multiple Rib Fractures. Due to Trauma. Causes Pain, Shortness of Breath. Diagnosis is Clinical. Management is O2, Possible Intubation, Possible Chest Tube. Pain control.

3. **Hemothorax:** If Large enough, Needs Drainage with a Chest Tube. If there is >200 mL/hour for the first two to four hours or > 1.5 L in the initial output then a Thoracotomy also needs to be done.

4. **Pericardial Tamponade:** Hypotension, Distant Heart Sounds, JVD. US FAST. Pericardiocentesis (if Nontraumatic). Needs Pericardial Window by Cardiothoracic Surgery. Thoracotomy if Penetrating injury with loss of Vital Signs in the ER or Cardiac Arrest Related.

5. **Pneumothorax**
    a. **Simple:** Chest Tube
    b. **Tension:** Needle Decompression, Chest Tube
    c. **Open:** Occlusive dressing with only 3 out of 4 sides Taped Closed. During this time, ensure that No Tension Pneumothorax develops. Definite Treatment is a Chest Tube.

6. **Cardiac Contusion**
    a. May present with Chest Pain, Shortness of Breath. Patient Needs Cardiac Monitoring if any evidence of EKG/Cardiac Enzymes abnormality or mechanism of injury is concerning. Also needs Echocardiogram and further Monitoring, Labs (Troponins), Repeat EKG's, etc. Consult Cardiology. Admit.

7. **Pulmonary Contusion**
    a. May present with Chest pain, Shortness of breath. Occurs Secondary to Trauma. Causes Edema, Bleeding in the Lung tissue. Diagnosis: Chest X-ray or CT Chest. Management: Oxygenation, Pain Medications, May need NPPV, Intubation. Avoid fluids if possible to avoid worsening of the Pulmonary Edema.

8. **Rib Fractures:** Diagnosis: Rib X-rays, CXR. Management: Oxygen. Pain Medications. Incentive Spirometer. Admit: Elderly Patients, More than One Rib Fracture. Comorbidities. Symptoms.

D. Skin

1. **Puncture Wound:** Irrigate the wound, Get X-ray to ensure No foreign bodies. Tetanus prophylaxis. Give Antibiotics for any wound that is contaminated or concerning. Also give Antibiotics with Pseudomonas coverage for Puncture Wound through the Sole of a Shoe

2. **Thermal Burn:**

   1. **First Degree Burn:** Painful Erythema of the Skin with solely Epidermal involvement
   Second Degree Burn: Painful Erythema, Bullae, Blister with Epidermal and Dermal involvement
   Third Degree Burn: All layers of the Skin are Involved. Loss of Sensation over Burn site, White

   "Rule of 9's": In an Adult, the head, neck is 9%, the front of the thorax is 18%, front and back of the thorax is 18%, each upper extremity is 9%, each lower extremity is 18%, the genitals are 1%.

   Any Singing of Facial Hair or Any Swelling of the Face or any Carbonaceous Sputum or any Signs of Shortness of Breath/Respiratory Distress/Stridor needs Early Intubation because these can all be indicative of Inhalation injury. Intubate early because the array can get edematous afterwards and much harder to intubate.

   Must consider Early Airway management. Needs Tetanus Shot. IV fluids: 2 to 4 mL/kg of Ringer Lactate per % TBSA Burned: Give First Half over first 8 hours and the rest over the next 16 hours (in a total 24 hour period). Consult Burn Center. Admit (If Severe burn, Moderate burn, Any burn of the Genitals, Hands, Feet, Any Joint or the Pelvic Region, Any evidence of Inhalation injury, Any Third Degree Burn, Lightning strike, Electrical burn, Chemical burn, Elderly patient, pediatric patient, trauma, Circumferential burn, any comorbidities, Any partial thickness burn with >10% TBSA: these patients all need to be sent to a Burn Center immediately!

3. **Bite wounds:** See Oral Boards Section. Needs Irrigation, Antibiotics, Tetanus Prophylaxis, X-ray. Consider Rabies Vaccination, based upon the animal that bit the patient and the region in the country/likelihood of rabies - See most current guidelines on CDC website

4. **High Pressure Injection Wounds:** These may seem benign but they are very dangerous because the material injects into the important interior regions (ie.

along the fascia, etc). Example: Paint guns: The paint goes into the fascia and other important structures. Pain, swelling. ischemia; Needs Stat Hand Surgeon/ Orthopedic Consult for OR repair (Surgical Debridement, etc.) and IV Antibiotics are also necessary. Tetanus Prophylaxis.

5. **Amputation of Digit:** If there is an amputated digit, wrap it in gauze that is soaked in saline and put this in a plastic bag. Then place the plastic bag in Ice water. However, **<u>Don't</u>** let the amputated digit itself touch any ice.

E. Head/Facial Trauma:

1. **Facial Fractures** (All of these need **Airway Assessment/Management** first)

2. **Le Fort Fracture:** Fracture of Midface. Type I: Upper teeth and Hard palate are Mobile. Type II: Nose and Palate are Mobile. Type III: The Whole Face is Mobile. Diagnosis: Clinical and Facial CT Scan. Airway Management. Needs IV Antibiotics, Stat Consult (Plastics/OMFS), Needs Surgery.

3. **Mandibular fracture:** Painful/Swelling of Jaw. X-ray. CT Facial Bones. Consult OMFS/ENT. Open Fracture Needs IV Antibiotics. Admit.

4. **Orbital Blowout Fracture:** Diplopia, Pain, Infraorbital Region Numbness (Upper Lip Numbness), Swelling, Enopthalmos. May have Inferior Rectus muscle trapped leading to eyeball looking straight upward. Needs stat Ophthalmology, OMFS/ENT Consult for Surgery. Give Antibiotics. Surgery.

5. **Septal Hematoma:** Must look in the Nare to see if there is evidence of Septal Hematoma (Mass along the septum). If so, needs Drainage and Anterior Nasal Packing, Antibiotics, ENT. If untreated, can lead to Septal Perforation and serious damage, loss of blood supply, etc.

6. **Basilar Skull Fracture:** Battle sign, Hemotympanum, Raccoon eyes, CSF Rhinorrhea, CSF Otorrhea. CT Head. Tx: Needs Antibiotics, Needs Stat Neurosurgery Consult.

7. **Nasal Fracture:** Often a Clinical Diagnosis. Needs Pain Medications, Ice, Follow Up with ENT

9. **Intracranial Injury:** Headache, Altered Mental Status, Possible Nausea, Vomiting. ie. Epidural Hematoma, Subdural Hematoma, etc. Needs Neurosurgery Consult

10. **Retrobulbar Hematoma:** After Trauma, Blood collects behind the Orbit. Proptosis, Ophthalmoplegia, Eye Pain. Stat Ophthalmology Consult. Needs Stat

Lateral Canthotomy. If Untreated, the patient can go blind.

11. Globe Rupture: After Trauma to the Globe. Subconjunctival Hemorrhage. Teardrop Pupil. Diagnosis is CT of the Orbit. Positive Siedel test. Management: Stat Ophthalmology Consult for Surgical Repair. IV Antibiotics. Shield the Eye and Don't let anything touch it.

F. C-Spine Trauma

1. Do a Thorough Neurological Examination. Always do imaging in anyone with trauma. Immobilize the C-spine if any concern for fracture. Patients who are Intoxicated, have a Distracting injury, Altered Mental Status, Focal Neurological Deficits or any Tenderness over the Cervical Spine need Immobilization of and Imaging of the C-spine. If the X-ray is negative but you have a high suspicion, do a CT or MRI. Any evidence of a C-Spine injury or fracture needs a Neurosurgery Consult. Unstable C-Spine Fractures: Jefferson Burst Fracture, Hangman Fracture, Dens Fracture Type II and III, Flexion Teardrop Fracture, Bilateral Facet Dislocation

G. GU Trauma

1. **Bladder Rupture:** Often manifests with Visible Hematuria, May also present with Pain over the Region of the Bladder. There are two types: Extraperitoneal and Intraperitoneal. Diagnosis is Retrograde Cystography or CT Cystography. Management is a Urology Consult for Surgery. Intraperitoneal Type needs Operative intervention.

2. **Genitalia:** Manifests with Pain, Swelling. Urology Consult for Operative Repair

3. **Penile Fracture:** Painful, Swollen and Limp. Rule out other injuries. Urology Consult. Needs Surgical Intervention.

4. **Renal:** May manifest with Hematuria Needs a CT Abdomen/Pelvis. This will need a Stat Urology Consult for Possible OR Repair or at the least, Observation

5. **Ureteral:** Manifests with Hematuria. Needs a CT Abdomen/Pelvis. This will need a Stat Urology Consult for Surgical Repair in the OR.

6. **Urethral:** Often occurs after an injury, for instance, a Bicycle/Horse-riding injury. Patient can present with a High Riding Prostate, Blood at the Urethral Meatus, Swelling of the External Genitalia, Hematuria. Diagnosis is a Retrograde Urethrogram. Management is a Stat Urology Consult for Surgical Repair in the OR. Reminder: Do **NOT** insert a Foley until you ensure that there is No urethral

injury, with A Retrograde Urethrogram. Consult Urology Stat for further Management.

H. Neck Trauma

1. Penetrating Zones
    1. **Zone III:** Above angle of mandible to base of head
    2. **Zone II:** Angle of mandible to cricoid
    3. **Zone I:** Cricoid to clavicle

2. **Vascular Neck Injuries:**

a. Any **Hard signs:** Thrill/Bruit, Expanding Hematoma, Lack of a Pulse, Bleeding. Hypotensive. Respiratory Distress: Needs immediate OR for Surgical Repair

b. If Soft signs (Hoarse voice, Crepitus/Subcutaneous Emphysema) needs CTA (if + needs OR) (If negative, consider Observation) (If Inconclusive, consider other modalities, like Bronchoscopy, EGD, etc.)

I. Pediatric Fractures/Dislocations

1. **Salter Harris:**
    1. **Type I:** Fracture through the Physis (Growth Plate) —> Orthopedic Follow Up
    2. **Type II:** Fracture through the Physis and Metaphysis —-> Orthopedic Follow Up
    3. **Type III:** Fracture through the Physis and Epiphysis —> Often Needs OR Repair. Consult Orthopedic
    4. **Type IV:** Fracture through the Physis, Metaphysis and Epiphysis —> Needs Immediate Orthopedic for OR Repair
    5. **Type V:** Compression Fracture in the Physis (Growth Plate) —> Needs Immediate Orthopedic for OR Repair

2. **Nursemaid's Elbow:** Child does not move the arm and holds it in a flexed and pronated position due to discomfort. Often occurs when the child's extended arm is pulled in an upward fashion. Radial Head Subluxation/Annular Head Displacement. Get x-ray if any History of trauma/Possibility of a Fracture. Management of Nursemaid's Elbow is either Supination and Flexion of the Elbow Or Hyperpronation and Extension of the Forearm. After either of these successful measures, the child starts using the Extremity again.

J. **Pelvic Fracture:** X-ray of Pelvis for the Diagnosis. A Pelvic fracture s/p trauma can lead to massive blood loss. Suspect in a Patient with an Unstable Pelvis and Unstable Vital Signs that's Unresponsive to Fluids. The patient may present

Tachycardic and Hypotensive. If Hypotensive, Give PRBC's. Needs Pelvic Binder and Stat Surgery Consult for the OR for Surgical Repair or with IR for Repair

K. Extremity Injuries:

1. Anterior Shoulder dislocation

Anterior: (The Images in the first row show an **Anterior Dislocation of the shoulder**)

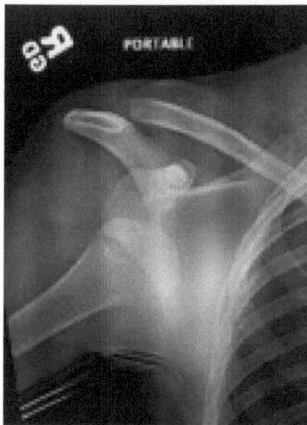

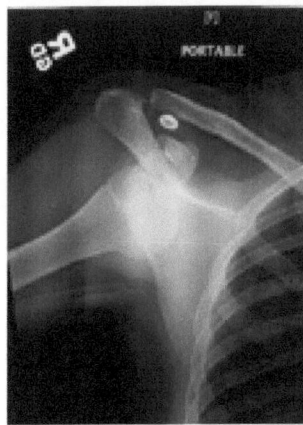

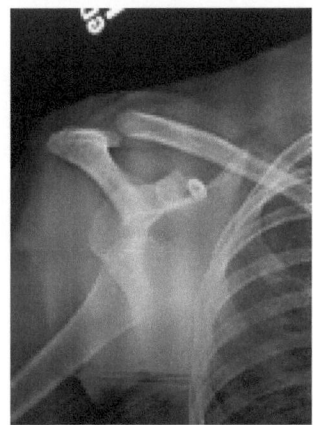

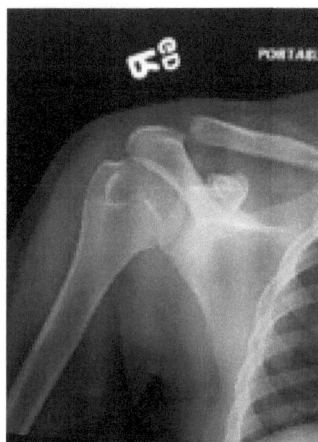

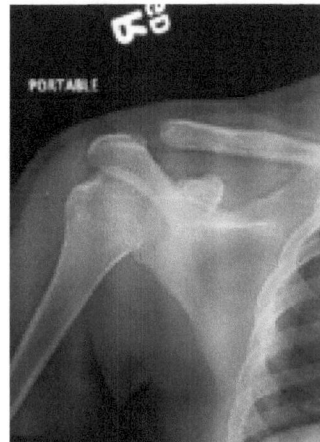

The images in the bottom row demonstrate the <u>relocation</u> of the anteriorly displaced shoulder joint after a single attempt at <u>reduction</u>, using the external rotation technique

2. **Posterior Shoulder Dislocation:** Often due to seizure or lightning strike. Patient is in pain and doesn't move shoulder in both anterior and posterior types of dislocation. Diagnosis is the X-ray. Management is Reduction (Axial Traction, External Rotation is the Method for Reduction). Traction-Countertraction. Get Post Reduction films and also Reassess Neurovascular Status Pre and Post Procedure

3. **Inferior Shoulder Dislocation:** The patient presents with the arm sticking out in an abducted position, with a flexed elbow and the hand is behind the head. Diagnosis is Clinical and X-ray. Management is: Axial Traction, Abduction. Simultaneously, Parallel Counter traction should be applied

4. Always do a thorough Neurological examination in these patients, both Pre and Post Reduction and always do X-rays, both Pre and Post Reduction

5. **Radius Fracture, Ulnar Fracture:**

a. **Monteggia Fracture:** Fractured Proximal Portion of the Ulna and Radial Head Displacement. Needs Stat Orthopedic Consult for ORIF

b. **Galeazzi Fracture:** Fracture of the Distal Radius with a Disrupted Radioulnar Joint. Needs Stat Orthopedic Consult for ORIF

6. **Radius Fracture**

a. **Colles Fracture:** Fracture of the Distal Radius is notable on Clinical Exam and X-ray. Orthopedic Consult dependent on the institution. Management is Reduction and a Sugar-Tong Splint. Prompt Orthopedic Follow Up

7. **Carpal Bone Fractures or Dislocations**

> a. **Scaphoid Fracture:** Clinical Diagnosis (May have Normal X-ray) Needs a Thumb Spica Splint. Of note: Often times, this does not show on Early X-ray/Imaging. If there is Tenderness over the Scaphoid region (Snuffbox Tenderness), Splint it (Thumb Spica Splint) and send it to Orthopedics! If Untreated, Complication is Avascular Necrosis. If Displaced, will need Stat Orthopedics for ORIF.

> b. **Lunate Fracture:** Diagnosis is Clinical and X-ray. Any tenderness over the Lunate bone needs a Thumb Spica Splint because this can also lead to Avascular Necrosis if it is not treated. Needs very close Orthopedic Follow Up

> c. **Lunate Dislocation:** Tender, Swollen. Diagnosis is Clinical, X-ray.

Treatment is Stat Orthopedic Consult for Immediate Closed Reduction or ORIF

d. **Perilunate Dislocation:** Tender, Swollen. Diagnosis is X-ray. Treatment is Stat Orthopedic Consult for Immediate Closed Reduction or ORIF

e. **Triquetrial Fracture:** Needs a Volar Splint and Orthopedic Follow Up. If Displaced: Needs Orthopedic for ORIF

8. Metacarpal Fracture

a. You should always be concerned that metacarpal fractures could be a fight bite. Did a humans teeth touch these bones? Is there a laceration? If so it is at very high risk of infection. Pain, swelling.
Patients are often embarrassed to admit this - when in doubt manage it this way! Xray, Tetanus shot, Stat Hand Surgeon/Orthopedic consult, IV Antibiotics, Splint, Admit

b. **Fifth Metacarpal Fracture = Boxer Fracture:** Fracture of the Neck of the 5th Metacarpal. Place an Ulnar Gutter Splint and Provide Orthopedic Follow Up as soon as possible, if Nondisplaced. If too much Angulation/Displacement, needs Orthopedic soon for Operative Repair

c. **First Metacarpal Fracture:**

   1) **Bennett Fracture** is an Intra-articular Fracture at the Base of the Thumb, with Subluxation of the CMC joint. It needs Orthopedic intervention for ORIF

   2) **Rolando Fracture** is an Intra-articular Fracture at the Base of the Thumb. It is a Comminuted Fracture. It needs Orthopedic intervention for ORIF.

9. Dislocation of the Knee

a. Needs Stat Orthopedic and Stat Vascular Surgery Consults

b. There is a Concern for issues with the Vasculature (ie Popliteal Artery) These Patients can have Arterial injuries, Nerve injuries

c. Diagnosis: Clinical, X-ray. Needs Angiography to ensure that there is No damage to the Popliteal artery (even if the knee popped back into place before the ER visit!)

    d. Management: Stat Orthopedic and Vascular Surgery Consult for any Neurovascular Issues

10. **Lisfranc Fracture:** X-ray will show Increased space between the 1st and 2nd Metatarsal and a Fracture at the Base of the 2nd Metatarsal. May palpate Tenderness and Visualize Bruising over the Midfoot Region. Needs Stat Orthopedic Consult for Operative Intervention.

11. **Open Fracture:** Needs Stat Orthopedics, IV Antibiotics and needs to be taken to the OR by the Orthopedic Surgeon

12. **Compartment Syndrome:** Increased Pain/Pressure in a Compartment of the Body, often times Extremities. Can occur after Trauma, etc. Painful, Tender, Paresthesias, Cold, Pale, Pulseless. Measure Compartment Pressure. Elevated in Compartment Syndrome. Needs Stat Orthopedic Consult. Needs OR (Fasciotomy).

13. **High-Pressure Injection:** i.e. Paint gun. These injuries can seem deceptively benign but are Very Dangerous. Needs a Stat Hand Surgery/Orthopedic Consult for OR for Surgical Debridement. IV Antibiotics.

14. **Calcaneus Fracture:** Can occur after jumping from a Height and these patients may subsequently present with Lower/Mid Vertebral Spine fractures. Calcaneus Fracture Diagnosis is on X-ray. Measure Boehler's Angle. Management is Surgical Intervention.

15. **Achilles Tendon Rupture:** Can feel the Palpable Tendon Rupture. Thompson Test Positive. Patient lays in the Prone Position and when the calf is Squeezed, it does Not Plantar flex. This is indicative of an Achilles Tendon Rupture.

16. **Hip Dislocation:** Diagnosis: X-ray or CT. Orthopedic Consult. Needs to Be Reduced immediately in order to Avoid Avascular Necrosis.

17. **Mallet Finger:** Finger (Distal portion: DIP) is Flexed secondary to some trauma. Management is to Splint the Finger (the DIP) in Extension for 6 to 8 weeks.

L. Multisystem Trauma

1. **Blast Injury:**

        a) **Primary** (Ears, Lungs, Intestines): Due to the Pressure from the Blast. ARDS, Air Embolism. Lung: Pulmonary Barotrauma. Dyspnea, Low O2, High RR, etc. Needs O2, Possible Intubation. Abdominal: Internal Hemorrhage. Ear: TM rupture

b) **Secondary** - Debris hits the person (Shrapnel wounds but notice that serious internal damage is possible)

c) **Tertiary** - Person is Thrown by Force (Can cause Blunt Injuries etc). Fractures/Loss of limbs etc.

d) **Quaternary** - All other injuries Secondary to the Blast that don't fall in the other categories. These include: Burn, Radiation, Crush injuries, etc.

e) Check for Radiation with the Detector, Remove and Dispose of Clothing in an Appropriate fashion/separate section where it won't be exposed to those who are uncontaminated

f) Must take care of the Airway! Treat any Immediate Trauma Concerns (ie Tension Pneumothorax, etc.)

g) Control Bleeding (Control with Pressure) i.e. on Extremities. Keep an eye out for Compartment Syndrome

h) Give Fluids, Blood Products. Imaging needed if Stable.
i.e. CXR, Pelvis X-ray, X-ray Extremity, CT scans, etc.

M. Questions to ask in a Motor Vehicle Collision

1. **Mnemonic: PLEASE**

Pain?

Loss of Consciousness?

Extricated?

Alcohol? Airbags Deployed? Ambulatory at the Scene?

Seatbelt on? Steering Wheel Damage? Speed?

Ejected?

Cases and Table Format to Review of the Oral Boards
Start familiarizing yourself with it now!

For the Oral Boards for Emergency Medicine, make sure that you have the following chart memorized so that you can draw it quickly, if you're given the time on the exam (or be able to recite it from memory, as you may not be given the time to draw out the entire chart). Ask all of these questions and review all of the potential cases (plus additional cases from additional review resources). If you have time, you can even think of a few on your own and practice with a friend. The oral boards are all about practicing systematically and repeatedly. Your encounters will often begin like this: You walk into the examination room and sit at the desk. You are handed a sheet and asked to start the case. You read the information stated (ie. "A 34 year old woman with Chest Pain") and have to start asking pertinent questions (this is where the chart created below is helpful). If you ask everything on this Chart and Know your Diagnostic/Management Principles, you will do well). Do this for all of your cases and you will do great. "Who is with the patient?" "Please ask them to stay." "May I have the vital signs"… "What do I hear, see and smell as I enter the room", etc. Good luck! You can do it!

Pre-Preparations for the layout of your sheet during the exam and topics to know for cases with information

1. Layout for How to Prepare for the Exam

2. Blank Sheet with the Figure of a man and sections to divide it into the following:

3. Reminder!! There are 6 vital signs!! Blood pressure, Heart rate, O2 sat, Respiratory rate, Temperature (Rectal temperature in infants/children) AND a Fingerstick Glucose!!

    1. The following shows you How to chart your oral boards review sheet and shows you what to memorize saying at the start of each encounter

    2. Everything that is listed from this point on, needs to be asked on Exam day, for each case!

    3. Who is with the patient? Please ask them to stay. (EMS, Family, etc.)

    4. VITAL SIGNS (6) BP__ HR __ O2 __ RR __ TEMP__ (ask for a RECTAL temperature ___ FSG (Fingerstick Glucose) ___

5. "What do I see, hear and smell when I walk into the room?"

6. **Nurse, Please Place Two Large Bore IV Lines in Both Antecubital Fossa, Place the patient on Oxygen and on a Cardiac Monitor. Also, please Repeat the vital signs after every intervention and every 5 minutes and report to me, thank you. Let's get a hold of any Old Records. While drawing the IV, please hold a full set of tubes. We can begin with sending off a CBC, CMP, PT/PTT, Type and cross and I will add onto this soon (ie EKG, Rhythm Strip, Troponins/CKMB/CK, Lactate, Lipase, ABG, Urinalysis, HCG (Pregnancy Test), CXR, CT, US etc).**

7. **Remember** to Continue to order the rest of the necessary **labs** in the primary survey along with **pertinent imaging!**

8. Introduce self to patient by his/her name and state your name. Ask whether the patient has any **allergies.**

9. The Table that you should follow is listed below:

Vital signs (6) BP ___ HR ___ O2 ___ RR ___ TEMP (peds rectal)___ FSG ___ *FSG: fingerstick glucose	"What do I see, hear, smell when I walk into the room?"	**Nurse, please place two large bore IV lines (in the antecubital fossa), place patient on O2 (via 2L), and on a Cardiac Monitor. Please hand me a rhythm strip and an EKG (as appropriate). Please repeat the vital signs Q5 minutes and report them to me, please. Thank you.**	Ask EMS, Family, etc to stay in the room because will have questions for them soon.
Primary Survey Airway Breathing Circulation Disability Exposure	**History** HPI PMH Allergies Medications Hospitalizations/ Surgeries Family history Occupation Sexual History Social History (Smoker, Alcohol, Drugs)	**Interventions** ie. IV lines, O2, Cardiac Monitor, NS, Pain Meds, Antibiotics, Antiemetics, IVF's, PRBC's, Tetanus Shot, Isolation, etc.	
Secondary Survey General HEENT Neck Chest Lungs Heart Back Abdomen Genitourinary Rectal Extremities Neurological Skin Lymph Nodes	**Labs and Imaging** ie. CBC, CMP, Lipase, PT/PTT, Type and screen, Cardiac enzymes (Troponin, CK, CK-MB), HCG, Urinalysis, Cultures EKG Rhythm Strip Chest Xray (Xray Pelvis, etc) CT scans (Head, C-S, Chest, Abdomen/Pelvis, etc.) Ultrasound (ie pregnancy, RUQ, US FAST...)	**Consults and Disposition** ie. Surgery, OBGYN, Cardiology, Neurosurgery, Neurology, GI, Orthopedics, Trauma, Ophthalmology, ENT, etc. ie. Admit or discharge (if discharging, provide follow up, instructions clearly explained, prescriptions, etc) MICU, SICU, PICU, OR, Floor, Telemetry bed, Cath Lab, etc.	

4. **Cases to Practice are listed below**

5. Think of possible EKG's on the exam (For Example: STEMI: ST elevations with reciprocal changes, Hyperkalemia with Peaked T waves or a Widened QRS Complex, Ventricular fibrillation, Ventricular Tachycardia, Torsades de Pointes, AV blocks, WPW, The Osborn "J" Waves of Hypothermia, Bradycardia, TCA overdose, Wellen's, Brugada, etc.) What CXR may present? (Tension PTX? Perforated viscous w/ free air?) What US may present? Positive US FAST with Free fluid? Cholecystitis? What CT scan may present? CT Head? Try to imagine all the scenarios that may present

6. CASE LIST

   1. Beta Blocker Overdose (A 60 year old man with fatigue)
      1. Often times in a depressed patient who overdoses on pills (AMS, Bradycardia, Hypotension, Hypoglycemia)
      2. Glucagon is the Treatment in addition to Cardiac Monitoring, Labs, etc.

   2. TCA Overdose (A 21 year old woman with a resolved seizure, but no prior hx of seizure)
      1. Anticholinergic syndrome (warm dry skin, constipation, urinary retention, mydriasis, dry mouth, possible confusion, tachycardia), possible seizure, hypotension, prolonged QT, Prolonged QRS, RBBB, dysrhythmias
      2. EKG needed (might see any of the following: widened QRS, deep s waves in I, avL, the R wave in avR's terminal portion has a ratio that is >3 mm in height
      3. Treatment: Sodium bicarbonate must be given in TCA Poisoning, Place on Cardiac Monitor, Give IVF's and Vasopressors if needed for Hypotension (ie Norepinephrine). For Seizure, give Lorazepam

   3. Aortic Dissection (A 55 year old man with back pain, severe)
      1. Pathophysiology: Tear in the wall of the Aorta leading to a False Lumen through which blood "dissects"
      2. RF's = Men, Smokers, HTN, Pregnancy, Marfan's, Ehler Danlos, Temporal Arteritis. Symptoms = Chest Pain, Back Pain, Abdominal Pain, Often Sudden Onset and Severe ("Tearing"), Radiates. Extremity Pain, Abdominal Pain, Often Hypertensive, Syncope, Can have CVA symptoms (Weakness, Slurred speech, Numbness etc). Syncope, Can present as an MI, CVA, Pulse Deficit, Mesenteric Ischemia, Ischemic Limb, CHF, Heart Block, Aortic Regurgitation (Murmur), Hoarseness, Horner syndrome, GI bleed, Dysphagia. Usually Hypertensive but can become hypotensive
      3. BP differential between the arms is possible. Pulses may not be normal between the extremities. Might hear aortic regurgitation murmur on exam. There may be neurological deficits present.
      4. Reminder: Reassess the patient often

5. Dx: Chest X-ray may show Widened Mediastinum and CTA Chest/Abdomen with IV Contrast (If patient is Stable) will show Aortic Dissection

6. What to order: CBC, CMP, PT/PTT, T&C, Lactate, D-dimer, UA, Cardiac enzymes, EKG, CXR, CT Chest/Abdomen (If Stable) or TEE (If Unstable)

7. Provide pain meds (ie morphine if not allergic); if hypertensive, either Labetalol or Esmolol (Beta blocker) first and then Nitroprusside (vasodilates). Given in this order to avoid reflex tachycardia that will worsen the dissection. If the patient is Hypotensive: IVFs, PRBCs, Stat OR

8. Stat Vascular Surgery Consult (Cardiothoracic Surgery) for Stat OR

4. **Abdominal Aortic Aneurysm (A 62 year old man with Back Pain):**
   1. Classic Scenario: Elderly man with Back Pain/Abdominal Pain/Syncope
   2. Risks: Smoking, Family History, Heart Disease, HTN
   3. Diagnosis: Ultrasound will show Enlarged Aorta but only CT scan will show if the Aorta is Ruptured. On Physical Exam, may feel a Pulsatile Abdominal Mass. Lower Extremity may have Decreased Pulses
   4. Weakness, Abdominal Pain, Back Pain, Syncope, Hip Pain, Hematuria
   5. CT Chest, Abdomen, Pelvis with IV Contrast if Stable. If Unstable (Can only see the presence of an AAA with an Ultrasound but Cannot see if it's ruptured or not)
   6. Stat Vascular Surgery Consult for Stat OR
   7. Often times, Hypotensive. Give IVF's, PRBC's. Do EKG, CXR, Send all Labs (CBC, CMP, PT/PTT, Cardiac Enzymes, D-Dimer, Lactate, UA, etc).

5. **Brugada's Syndrome**
   1. Heart Disorder that can cause Sudden Cardiac Death
   2. Type I: Looks like a Humpback ST Elevation in at least two leads within V1-V3 and the T wave is inverted. There is a RBBB pattern.
   3. Can present with Palpitations, Syncope, Dizziness, Near Syncope, Family History of Early Cardiac Death
   4. Treatment is AICD

6. **Wellen's Syndrome**
   1. Critical stenosis of the Proximal LAD
   2. Deep T wave inversions or biphasic T waves in leads V2, V3
   3. Often Cardiac Cath shows 100% or Severe Occlusion of the LAD
   4. Treatment is Admission and Early Cath Lab for Revascularization or else patient has High Risk of MI and Death

7. **STEMI:**
    1. **STEMI'S Best Management is Timely PCI in the Cath Lab!**
    2. Septal: V1, V2 (STE)
    3. Anterior: V3, V4 (STE)
    4. Anteroseptal: V1, V2, V3, V4 (STE)
    5. Lateral: I, avL, V3, V4 (STE). Reciprocal Changes (STD): II, III, aVF
    6. Anterolateral: I, aVL, V3, V4, V5, V6 (STE). Reciprocal Changes: II, III, aVF
    7. Inferior: II, III, aVF (STE), Reciprocal changes (STD): I, aVL (Do a Right sided EKG to see if Right ventricular infarction)
    8. Posterior: ST Depressions (Reciprocal changes) in V1, V2, V3 (Need to also do Posterior leads EKG of V7, V8, V9)

8. **STEMI (Anterior) - A 48 year old man with Chest Pain: Needs Cath Lab stat!**

9. **STEMI (Inferior): IVF's and cath lab; do Right sided EKG to see if RVI - A 40 year old woman with chest pain**
    1. Do Right sided EKG (V3R, V4R) where you will see ST Elevations
    2. What medications are contraindicated in this patient? Anything that decreases preload (Nitroglycerin, Morphine, Vasodilators, Diuretics are **CONTRAINDICATED!** Never use these) Why? These patients are preload dependent!
    3. What should you give these patients? IV Fluids (NS), Aspirin, Cath Lab STAT

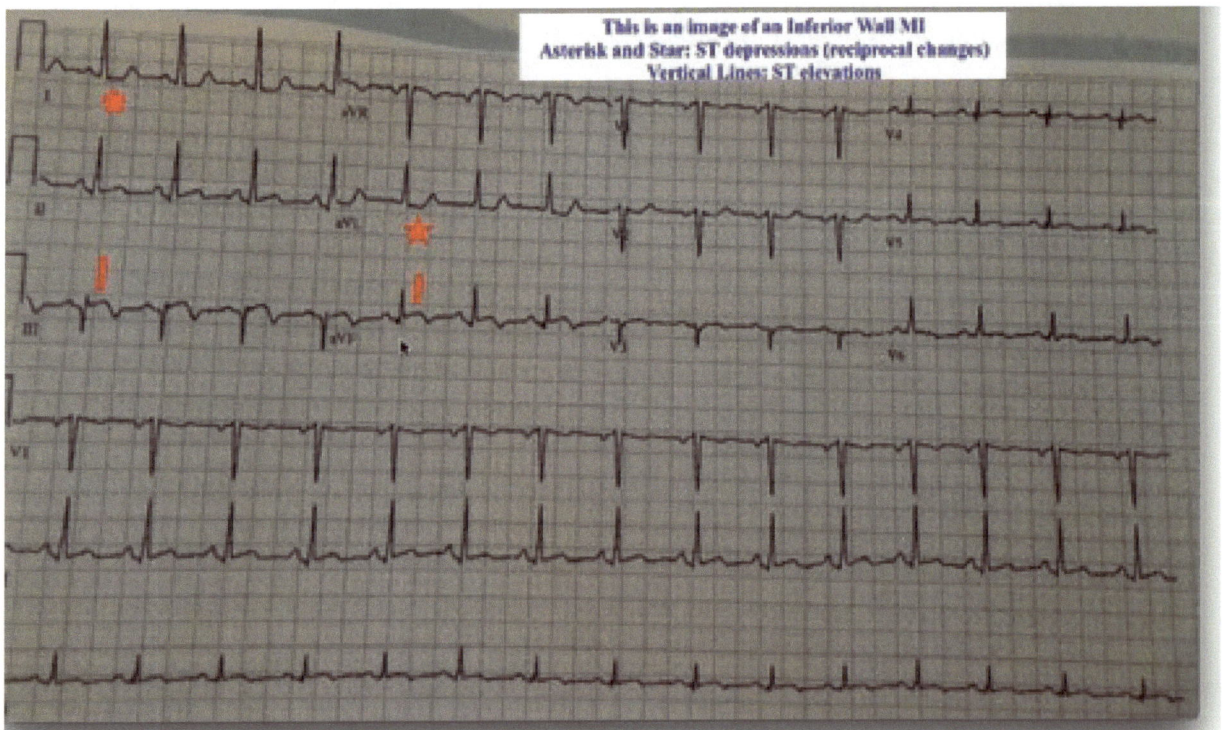

This is an image of an Inferior Wall MI
Asterisk and Star: ST depressions (reciprocal changes)
Vertical Lines: ST elevations

Note: The patient with this EKG had a 100% Occlusion of the Right coronary artery. Note that there is an Inferior Wall MI notable in this EKG

Now imagine any other STEMI and you will see similar or even more pronounced changes in the sections discussed above, depending on the type of STEMI.

10. **STEMI (Posterior): ST Depressions V1, V2, V3? Look at V7-V9 leads to see ST Elevations - A 40 year old man with Cough, Chest pain**
    1. EKG shows **Horizontal ST Depressions** in V1, V2, possibly V3. Tall R waves, Upright T waves (usually), R wave usually taller than S wave or the same size. At this point you need to do another EKG to look at the Posterior Leads: V7, V8, V9, which will show ST elevations. This needs to go to the Cath lab STAT as all STEMIs (PCI).

11. **Pulmonary Embolism - A 22 year old woman with Dyspnea**
    1. Chest Pain, Dyspnea, Leg Pain/Swelling, Tachycardia
    2. Well's criteria: DVT symptoms, Hx of Malignancy, Hemoptysis, Prior PE or DVT, Immobilization or Surgery or Long Travel in the past one month, Heart Rate >100, OCP use, Family History of Blood Disorders, Obesity, CHF
    3. CTA Chest (If Renal Failure, do a V/Q scan instead)
    4. Note: A D-dimer can only help to rule out PE in a LOW risk patient. It is **NOT** useful in a Moderate to High risk patients. Nevertheless, If you suspect it, Scan it.
    5. Treatment: Anticoagulation (ie. Lovenox or Heparin)

12. **Simple Pneumothorax - A 17 y/o man with Dyspnea**
    1. Diagnosis: Clinical and Chest X-ray. Absent Breath Sounds Unilaterally, Hyperresonance. Pneumothorax on Chest X-ray (Absent lung markings leading to edge, etc). Ultrasound with Linear probe can show Absence of Lung sliding and "Stratosphere sign" for Pneumothorax.
    2. Treatment = Chest Tube

13. **Cardiac Tamponade - A 33 y/o patient with Dyspnea and Chest Pain**
    1. JVD, Muffled Heart Sounds, Hypotension, Pulses Paradoxes. EKG may show Electrical Alterans
    2. Treatment = Pericardiocentesis (if Unstable) and Definitive Management is Cardiology/Cardiothoracic Surgery Consult for a Pericardial Window

14. **Deep Vein Thrombosis (DVT) - A 35 year old man with Leg pain**
    1. Risk factors: Recent Immobilization (ie Recent Surgery/Hospitalization, Long Plane/Car Rides, etc), Personal or Family History of DVT or PE or Hereditary blood disorders (Thrombophilias), Pregnancy, OCP use, Obesity, History of a Malignancy

2. Diagnosis: Ultrasound Doppler Lower Extremity Venous
3. Treatment: Anticoagulation (ie. Lovenox or Heparin initially)

15. **Tension Pneumothorax - A 33 y/o man s/p Trauma**
    1. JVD, Deviated Trachea, Unilateral Absent Breath Sounds, Hyperresonance
    2. Treat with Needle Decompression before CXR if Suspecting Tension Pneumothorax and then place a Chest Tube
    3. Scenarios: s/p Trauma, a patient who is intubated and taken in a helicopter (air pressure changes)

16. **Necrotizing Fasciitis - A 50 y/o with leg pain**
    1. "Pain out of Proportion" to Physical Exam Findings
    2. May find Bullae, Discoloration, Crepitus, Drainage, Swelling, Redness
    3. Treatment: Stat Surgical Consultation for Debridement, IVF's and IV Antibiotics

17. **Ovarian Torsion - A 30 y/o with Abdominal Pain**
    1. Twisting of the Ovary leading to Decreased Blood Supply and thereby potential loss of function of the organ along with loss of fertility if not corrected promptly
    2. Lower Abdominal Pain, Nausea, Vomiting
    3. Ultrasound Transvaginal with Doppler imaging
    4. Needs to go stat to the OR. Stat OBGYN Consult. If the Ultrasound is Negative but you are still concerned for Torsion presenting with Torsing/Detorsing, Admit to the OBGYN (Stat Consult) for OR

18. **Pelvic Inflammatory Disease (PID) - A 17 y/o with Abdominal Pain**
    1. In young patients, generally sexually transmitted. Usually caused by chlamydia trachomatis, neisseria gonorrheae or trichomonas vaginalis (sometimes multiple and always treat like coexisting together).
    2. Abdominal Pain, Pelvic Pain, Fever, Vaginal discharge, Possible STD History/Exposure, Adnexal Tenderness, CMT (Cervical Motion Tenderness)
    3. US Transvaginal w Doppler to r/o TOA, torsion, etc.
    4. Management is: Azithromycin, Ceftriaxone, Metronidazole
    5. Consider Admission if: Toxic (Fever, N/V are uncontrolled), Possibly other diagnosis thats equally or more severe, Pregnancy, TOA also present, Failed Outpatient Treatment, Unreliable follow up. In these cases IV Antibiotics are needed and so is Admission

19. **Tubo-Ovarian Abscess (TOA) - A 22 y/o with Abdominal Pain**
    1. Abscess of the ovary or fallopian tube or the ligament surrounding it
    2. Abdominal Pain, Nausea, Vomiting, Fever, Pelvic Pain, Vaginal discharge
    3. Adnexal Tenderness, CMT tenderness

4. Diagnosis: Ultrasound
5. Treatment: IV Antibiotics, Stat OBGYN Consult, Possible Surgery, Drainage
6. Admit

20. Ectopic pregnancy - A 40 y/o with Vaginal Spotting
1. Pregnancy is situated outside the uterus (ie in the fallopian tube) and therefore not viable
2. Abdominal Pain and or Vaginal Bleeding or Spotting
3. Send BHCG quantitative and Ultrasound Transvaginal in addition to usual Labs, PT/PTT, Rh, Type & Cross
4. Stat OBGYN Consult and Admit
5. Stable: Methotrexate (If Not Contraindicated)
6. Unstable: OR for Lap

21. Meningitis- A 22 y/o with a Headache
1. Headache, Photophobia, Neck stiffness, Fever/chills, Nausea, Vomiting, Lethargy
2. Labs, PT/PTT, UA, Blood cultures, CT Head (ie. Focal Neurological Deficits, Seizure, Possible Brain Mass, Papilledema, History of Brain issues, Elderly Patient, Immunocompromised, Any Concern for a Mass Lesion, which would be a Contraindication to an LP), Lumbar puncture (CSF studies: Cell count with Differential, Culture, Gram Stain, Glucose, Protein)
3. IV Antibiotics and Dexamethasone (Steroids). Steroids should only be given in Older infants, children and adults but **Not** in young infants (**Not** in neonates). Treat right when you suspect it but send Blood Cultures first (Note: Young Infants and Elderly need Listeria coverage with Ampicillin). < 1 month get: Ampicillin + Cefotaxime (may consider Ampicillin + Gentamicin). 1 month to 3 months: Ampicillin + Cefotaxime. > 3 months: Ceftriaxone + Vancomycin
4. Admit

22. Eclampsia - A 30 y/o woman with Elevated BP Reading
1. Seizure + Preeclampsia (Think of Eclampsia in a pregnant or postpartum woman with a Seizure)
2. Treat both Preeclampsia and Eclampsia the same: Prevent/Treat Seizure with Magnesium, Control BP if high with Labetalol or Hydralazine and get an OBGYN Consult Stat for Immediate Delivery

23. Subarachnoid Hemorrhage - A 44 y/o with a Headache

1. Headache, Nausea, Vomiting, Neck Stiffness, Photophobia
2. Diagnosis is CT Head Noncontrast. If there is a Negative CT head, then can do Lumbar puncture (if No contraindications) which generally shows Bloody Tap throughout all 4 tubes and Xanthochromia (s/p Centrifuge)
3. Stat Neurosurgery consult
4. Give Nimodipine (Prevents Vasospasm that is caused by SAH)

24. Ventricular Tachycardia - A 22 y/o with Palpitations

1. Pulseless Ventricular Tachycardia: Immediate Defibrillation (and follow latest ACLS guidelines) (No pulse)
2. Torsades (Polymorphic Vtach) also needs Defibrillation (360 J monophonic or 200 J biphasic). Should also give Magnesium
3. Pulse present but Hemodynamically Unstable (ie Chest Pain, Hypotension, AMS etc). Needs Synchronized Cardioversion (Adults: 100 J)
4. Stable needs Amiodarone 150 mg bolus over 10 minutes and then a drip (1 mg/min x 6 hours) (Asymptomatic or Mild Symptoms like Palpitations)
5. Admit to Cardiology (CCU)

25. CVA - A 60 y/o man with Numbness in left hand

1. Time of onset, Symptoms, Neurological exam. CT Head. Labs (CBC, CMP, PT/PTT, Cardiac enzymes/Troponin, Pregnancy test (women), CXR, EKG)
2. Needs Physical exam (including Neurological exam), CT Head Noncontrast Stat
3. Neurology Consult Stat (Stroke team)
4. If within a window of 3 hours (in some patients, up to 4.5 hours guidelines), depending on symptoms (ie symptoms worsening, significant deficits on NIHSS stroke score, Negative CT Head, If there is a higher chance of long term disability if not given, Patient is within the appropriate time window, No Contraindications present etc.) Consult with Neurology on decision for tPA (Ensure that No contraindications exist prior to Administration!)
5. Admit, Neurology Consult

26. Renal Colic - A 30 y/o man can't sit still due to Flank Pain

1. "Writhing" in pain. Flank pain, Possible Nausea, Vomiting
2. CT Abdomen/Pelvis Noncontrast, Urinalysis, Labs, HCG
3. IVF's. Pain Meds. Urologist
4. When to Discharge and When to Admit (ie Obstructed, UTI and Kidney stone, Elderly, Pregnancy, Unreliable follow up, Size of the stone is > 5 mm in size, Single Kidney, Comorbidities, Infection, etc.)

27. **Pericarditis - A 35 year old woman with Chest pain**
    1. Inflammation of the Pericardial lining. Fever possible, Chest Pain.
    2. Diffuse ST elevations, PR Depressions (Except in aVR, in which there is generally ST Depression and PR elevation)
    3. Pericardial Friction Rub is Possibly Audible
    4. Chest Pain improves with Leaning Forward and Worsens in the Supine Position. Worsens with Breathing
    5. Management: NSAID
    6. Note: Also send off Cardiac Enzymes. Needs: Echocardiogram, Cardiology consult, Admit if any concern for another etiology (ie MI), effusion or tamponade present, febrile, comorbidities, immunocompromised, recent trauma, on warfarin, etc.

28. **Child Abuse - A Bruised 2 month old child, parents say he rolled off the bed**
    1. Look for a pattern of injury that is inconsistent with the child's age and do physical exam, imaging (ie. A 4 month old with a fracture that parent says patient "rolled off the bed")

29. **Alcohol withdrawal, DT's - A Known Alcoholic presents with AMS, Tremor**
    1. Tremor, Seizure, Delirium/AMS, Tachycardia, Anxious, Palpitations. Airway Management. Send Labs (CBC, CMP, Fingerstick glucose), CT Head (to R/O Hemorrhage from trauma). Give Benzodiazepine (ie. Lorazepam). Give Thiamine, Glucose (if low). Admit to ICU!

30. **Carotid Artery Dissection - A 38 y/o with Dysarthria**
    1. Often times the Cause of Stroke in Young People Under age 45
    2. Occurs Spontaneously or after Trauma (can happen after a massage to the neck etc). Blood enters Artery and Thrombosis can form, leading to a Stroke, SAH, Pseudoaneurysm etc.
    3. Headache, Neck Pain, Eye Pain, Neurological Deficits, CVA (Dysarthria, Aphasia, Weakness, Visual Changes/Loss, etc.), Horner's Syndrome (Ptosis, Miosis)
    4. Dx CT Head and then a CTA or MRA
    5. Tx: Extracranial Dissection: Anticoagulation, Surgery
    6. Tx: Intracranial Dissection: Endovascular Surgery (Neurosurgery) (Anticoagulation is CONTRAINDICATED!!)
    7. Reminder: If there is any Intracranial extension of the dissection, Anticoagulation is **CONTRAINDICATED!**

31. **Vertebral Artery Dissection - A 40 y/o with Ataxia**
    1. Often times the cause of Stroke in young people under age 45
    2. Headache, Neck Pain, Ataxia, Nausea, Vomiting, Neurological Deficits, CVA symptoms (Weakness, Aphasia, Dysarthria, Visual Loss, etc), Vertigo, Double Vision
    3. Dx: CT Head and then CTA or MRA
    4. Tx: Anticoagulation
    5. If there is any Intracranial extension of the Dissection, Anticoagulation is CONTRAINDICATED!

32. **Cavernous Sinus Thrombosis - A 30 y/o with Headache**
    1. Blood Clot in the Cavernous Sinus that is usually due to an Infection
    2. Eye Pain, Headache, Fever, Nausea, Vomiting, Photophobia (and other Meningeal Signs), Lethargy/AMS, Sepsis, Papilledema, Exophthalmos, Cranial 3, 4, 6 Nerve Palsies (Cannot move Extra Ocular Muscles), Infraorbital or Periorbital Edema, Ptosis, Proptosis, Chemosis, Decreased Visual Acuity, Possible Injected Conjunctiva
    3. Diagnosis: CT Head, MRI, MRV, Lumbar Puncture (If No contraindications)
    4. Needs IV Antibiotics, Steroids, Neurology, Neurosurgery Consultation, ICU, Ophthalmology

33. **Heat Stroke - A 27 y/o with AMS and a Temperature of 107 after running a marathon**
    1. Can be Exertional (ie. Young people exercising in the heat) or Nonexertional (Elderly people)
    2. High Body Temperature (ie 105 and above, often)
    3. Order: CBC, CMP, FSG, ABG, CK level. Note look at LFT's, Renal Functioning, Potassium carefully as they may be Very Elevated. EKG, CXR, CT Head
    4. Often times doesn't sweat. May have Altered Mental Status
    5. Can cause Multiorgan Failure
    6. Life Threatening!
    7. Cool Immediately (Cooling with Water, Fan, Ice Packs). Airway Management, Hydration. If Seizure, give Benzodiazepine. Admit for Monitoring and Repeat Tests/Labs, etc.

34. **Mesenteric Ischemia - A 62 y/o woman with Atrial fibrillation and Severe Abdominal Pain**
    1. Etiologies: Arterial Embolus, Arterial Thrombosis, Non-flow/Low flow state, Venous Thrombosis
    2. "Pain Out of Proportion to exam" (Patient feels severe pain even if the Exam is Benign)
    3. Abdominal Pain (Severe), Nausea, Vomiting, Diarrhea

4. Often the Patient has Atrial Fibrillation (or some Cardiac Disease), CAD, CHF, Elderly Patient, Valvular issues of the Heart
    1. CBC, CMP, PT/PTT, Type & Screen, Lactate (Increased), Increased Anion Gap, Labs, Cardiac Enzymes (Troponins), CTA Abdomen/Pelvis, EKG, CXR
5. IVF's, IV Antibiotics, Papaverine, **Stat Surgery Consult** for ie. Surgical Embolectomy, Thrombectomy, Stent, Resection, etc by Surgery, IR, Vascular Surgery. The prior mentioned treatments will be conducted depending on the underlying etiology.

35. **Small Bowel Obstruction (SBO) - A 60 y/o man with Abdominal Pain**
    1. Patient has Abdominal Pain, Nausea, Vomiting, Constipation
    2. X-ray Abdomen Flat and Erect, CT Abdomen/Pelvis
    3. Stat Surgery Consult, NG tube if Vomiting and No contraindications to it, IVF's

36. **Dialysis patients and complications**
    1. Hyperkalemia (see # 37)
    2. Volume Overload: Shortness of Breath
    3. Cardiac Tamponade
    4. Bleeding access site
    5. Coagulopathy (since platelet dysfunction)
    6. MI
    7. Infection
    8. GI Bleed or other bleeds (ie CNS)

37. **Hyperkalemia - A 32 y/o Dialysis patient with Weakness, who missed his last Hemodialysis**
    1. EKG findings as levels progressively increase: Peaked T waves, PR Interval increases, P waves may disappear, QRS widens, Sine wave, Vfib, Asystole
    2. Possible symptoms: Palpitations, Fatigue, Weakness, Numbness, Dyspnea, Nausea/Vomiting, Chest Pain
    3. Treatment: Calcium Gluconate (Slow infusion), Regular Insulin 10 units, D50, Albuterol Nebulizer, Sodium Bicarbonate (1 amp), Kayexalate 30 grams PO
    4. Key point: Who is Calcium contraindicated in? Contraindicated in Patients who are on Digoxin
    5. **Mnemonic: Treatment for Hyperkalemia: C I c(see) a BAD K = C**alcium gluconate, **I**nsulin, **B**icarbonate, **A**lbuterol, **D**extrose, **K**ayexalate

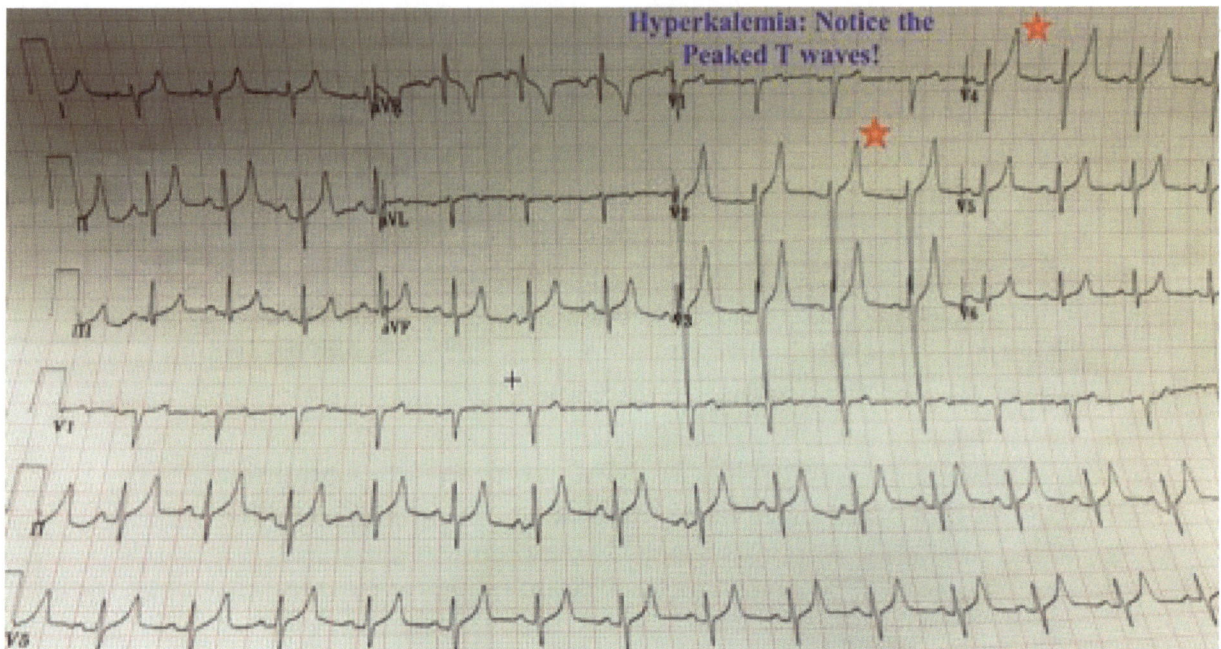

Hyperkalemia: Notice the Peaked T waves!

38. **Intussusception - A 2 y/o child is Lethargic and Cries intermittently, while drawing his legs up towards his abdomen**
    1. Intestines coil in or "Telescope" in on themselves
    2. Abdominal Pain (Pediatric often 3 months to 2 years old). Often draw legs to abdomen. Vomiting, Currant Jelly Stools, Sausage Mass Possible.
    3. Ultrasound Abdomen. Note: Air Enema can be Diagnostic and Treatment.
    4. Interventional Radiology (Generally Contrast enema (Air enema) given) and Consult Surgery initially, in the event of failure to reduce or perforation).

39. **Appendicitis - A 25 y/o woman with periumbilical pain yesterday, RLQ today**
    1. Periumbilical pain, RLQ pain, can even be Generalized Abdominal Pain, Nausea, Vomiting, Loss of Appetite. Possible Exam with McBurney's Point Tenderness, Rovsing sign, Psoas sign, Obdurator sign
    2. CT Abdomen/Pelvis (Consider Ultrasound in children if available at facility)
    3. Stat Surgery Consult, NPO, IVF's, IV Antibiotics

40. **Thyroid Storm - A 26 y/o patient with Palpitations**
    1. **Mnemonic** (sorry, this one stretches it a bit!): During the (Thyroid) *STORM*, **PAWS** (the puppy) - **PATS** - **SHADE** (the kitten) on the back to comfort her, Both **C**uties **H**ave **F**ur
    2. **P**alpitations, **A**nxious, **W**eakness, **W**eight loss, **P**roptosis, **A**ltered mental **S**tatus, **T**remor, **T**hyroid Mass, **T**achycardia, **S**weating, **S**hortness of **B**reath, **H**ypermetabolic state, **H**eat intolerance, **A**nxiety, **A**trial Fibrillation, **D**iarrhea, **E**dema (pulmonary, periorbital, pretibial), **C**HF (Congestive heart **F**ailure), **H**ypertension, **F**ever

3. Send CBC, CMP, Cardiac Enzymes (Troponin, etc), ABG, TSH, free T3, free T4, Pro-BNP, UA, CXR, EKG; For Purposes of Management, the Diagnosis is Clinical (send off Thyroid levels as well: TSH, free T4, free T3; but remember these take hours to come back so if clinically suspected, treat!)
4. Management:
    1. **Mnemonic: PAID = PTU, Propranolol, Antibiotics (if infection is the underlying cause), Airway, Iodide, Dexamethasone**
        1. Airway Management
        2. Propranolol or Esmolol (Beta blocker): Decreases the sympathetic symptoms
        3. Propylthiouracil (PTU): Blocks thyroid hormone production or Methimazole: Blocks thyroid hormone production
        4. Potassium Iodide (SSKI): Only <u>give Iodide at least one hour after</u> PTU or methimazole to prevent the release of thyroid hormone. Potassium Iodide Blocks the release of thyroid hormone
        5. Steroids (Dexamethasone): Doesn't allow T4 to cover to T3 peripherally and treats any concomitant adrenal insufficiency
        6. Give IVF's, Treat Underlying Cause, If Hyperthermia, Cool the patient

41. **Hemolytic Uremic Syndrome (HUS)**
    1. **Mnemonic: DART or ART or TAR or RAT can be used as Mnemonics!**
    2. Often preceded by Diarrhea (Ecoli 0157:H7)
    3. **Anemia**
    4. **Renal Failure**
    5. **Thrombocytopenia**
    6. Consult Hematology and usually supportive care (**<u>Never</u>** give antibiotics because it can worsen the HUS)

42. **Thrombotic Thrombocytopenic Purpura TTP - A 32 y/o with Confusion, Fever and Abnormal Labs**
    1. **Mnemonic: NO FART**
    2. **Neurological (AMS, Seizure, etc.)**
    3. **Fever**
    4. **Anemia**
    5. **Renal failure**
    6. **Thrombocytopenia**
    7. Management: Consult Hematology and Management is Plasmapheresis
    8. Note: You don't have to have all of the above to make it a diagnosis, so keep it in the differential

43. **Hypertensive Emergency -**
    1. A 60 y/o with a BP of 200/110 and a Headache
    2. A woman with an Elevated BP, who is 4 weeks Postpartum and just had a Seizure (Eclampsia)
    3. **Mnemonic: CHAPERONES**
    4. **C**ongestive Heart Failure - Leg Swelling Bilaterally, DOE, PND, Orthopnea, Dyspnea
    5. **C**VA (Thrombotic, Hemorrhagic) - Headache, Weakness, Focal Deficits, Dysarthria, etc.
    6. **I**ntracranial **H**emorrhage - Headache, Nausea, Vomiting
    7. **A**cute **C**oronary Syndrome (Myocardial Infarction) - Chest pain, possible generalized weakness, nausea, vomiting, diaphoresis
    8. **A**ortic Dissection - Chest pain, Back Pain, Possible CVA symptoms (Weakness, Focal Deficits), Abdominal Pain (mesenteric ischemia), Leg Pain, Dysphagia, GI Bleeding, Hoarse Voice
    9. **P**reeclampsia, Eclampsia - Hypertension in Pregnancy, Edema, Seizure
    10. **A**cute **P**ulmonary Edema - Shortness of breath, DOE, PND, Orthopnea
    11. **A**cute **R**enal failure - Decreased urine, Weakness, Nausea, Vomiting
    12. Hypertensive **E**ncephalopathy - Headache, AMS, Seizure, Nausea, Vomiting, HTN, Visual changes
    13. **S**ubarachnoid hemorrhage - Headache, Nausea, Vomiting, Neck Stiffness, Photophobia

44. **Status Epilepticus - A Patient who is persistently seizing without return to baseline (An Emergency)**
    1. Seizure lasting for more than 5 minutes without return to baseline level of alertness/consciousness. Assess Airway. Consider Airway Management.
    2. Place Two Large Bore IV lines, Oxygen, Cardiac Monitor
    3. Intubate the patient
    4. Benzodiazepines (Lorazepam) are first line
    5. If not working, consider Phenytoin
    6. Send Fingerstick Glucose (FSG), Labs/Studies (CBC, CMP, Toxicology screen, EKG, UA, ABG, Pregnancy Test etc).
    7. Think of whether this is due to an Infection (Meningitis), etc. Consider CT Head, etc.
    8. Neurology Consult, Needs Admission

45. **Hypoglycemia - A Woman with Lethargy, FSG is 25**
    1. Weakness, Lethargy, Confusion/AMS. Always check a FSG Stat!
    2. Fingerstick Glucose and if Hypoglycemic, the Treatment is Dextrose
    3. If the Hypoglycemia is due to Sulfonylurea, give Dextrose, Octreotide and Admit

4. If the Hypoglycemia is due to Sulfonylurea or a Moderate to Long acting Insulin, Admit because the half lives are long and can lead to Rebound Hypoglycemia

46. **GBS (Guillain Barre) Syndrome - A woman with Weakness in the Legs**
    1. <u>Mnemonic: GAIN</u> = GBS, Ascending Paralysis, Airway, IVIG, ICU, Neurology Consult
    2. Ascending Weakness/Ascending Paralysis
    3. Can occur after Viral Syndrome
    4. CSF may show dissociation of protein and abcs (High Protein in CSF with a Normal Cell Count)
    5. Treatment: Airway, IVIG, Neurology consultation, Admit, ICU

47. **RMSF (Rocky Mountain Spotted Fever) - A 15 y/o with a Rash who recently visited the Southeast portion of the United States of America**
    1. Recent visit to area with possible ticks
    2. Fever, Headache, Rash (Starts on Wrists, Ankles and then moves Centrally (to Trunk) and then it goes to Palms and Soles), Fatigue, Muscle Aches, Possible Nausea, Vomiting, Possible Conjunctivitis
    3. Treatment: Doxycycline

48. **Peritonsillar Abscess - A 30 y/o with a sore throat and hoarseness**
    1. Fever, Sore throat, Drooling, Hoarseness, Throat pain, Difficulty swallowing
    2. One Tonsil Larger, Erythematous, Uvula Deviated to the Opposite side
    3. ENT, Needle Aspiration and IV Antibiotics

49. **Retropharyngeal Abscess - A 20 y/o with a Sore Throat and Odynophagia**
    1. Sore Throat, Fever, Neck Pain, Painful Swallowing, Difficulty Swallowing
    2. CT Neck and Chest
    3. IV Antibiotics
    4. Stat ENT Consult

50. **Temporal Arteritis - A 60 y/o with a Headache**
    1. Usually in Elderly (>50)
    2. Polymyalgia Rheumatica precedes it usually
    3. Headache (in Temporal Region), Fatigue, Jaw Claudication, Weakness, can cause Blindness, Visual Loss if untreated
    4. ESR high (>50)
    5. Treatment: Give Steroids and Admit and Consult Ophthalmology
    6. Definitive Diagnosis is Temporal Artery Biopsy (but if Suspected, Give Steroids before this!)

51. Septic Arthritis - A 20 y/o with a Swollen, Warm Knee Joint
1. Infection of the Joint. Painful joint
2. Erythema, Warmth, Swelling and Tenderness of the Region at the joint
3. Diagnosis: Arthrocentesis and Analysis of Fluid
4. Management: Antibiotics and Stat Orthopedic Consult and Admit

52. Prolonged QT and Torsades

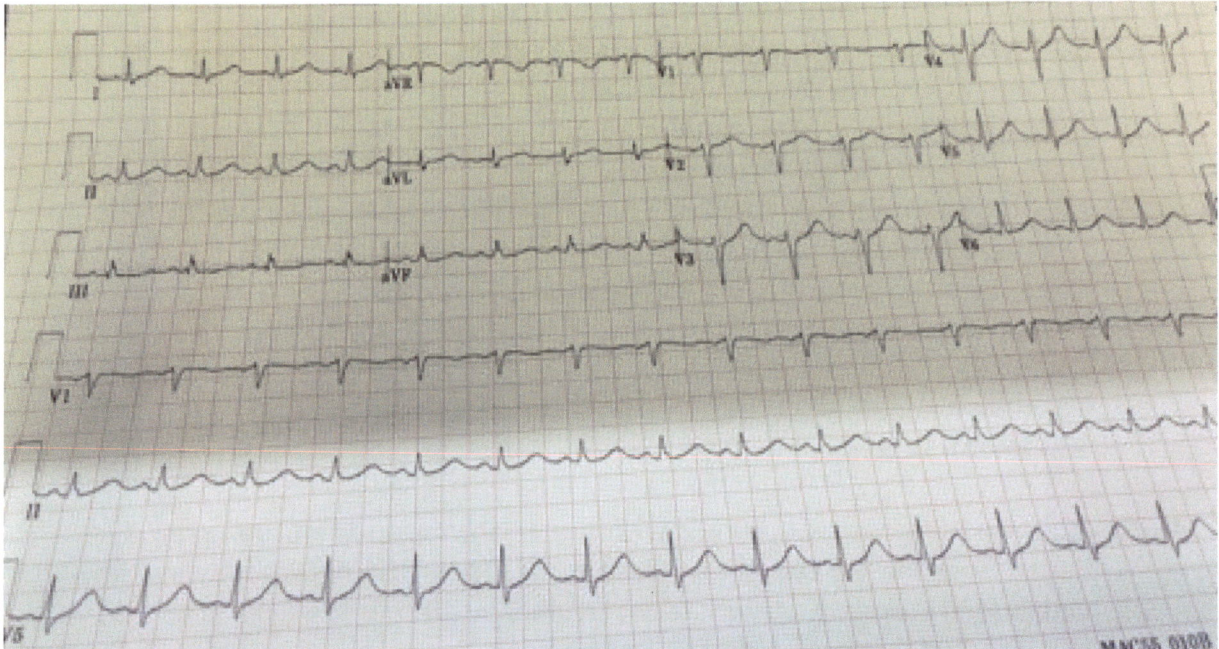

1. EKG: Prolonged QT EKG. Prolonged QT has many causes, including medications that prolong the QT, congenital issues, electrolyte disorders etc.

Note: If a patient has Torsades de Pointes, it is considered Polymorphic Tachycardia. It is often caused by a Prolonged QT interval. It is managed with Defibrillation and Magnesium! Admit to CCU! Cardiology consult

53. Tylenol overdose - A 20 y/o overdosed on Tylenol and has Nausea, vomiting
1. Labs (CBC, CMP, PT/PTT, Type, Lipase, Toxicologic studies), Acetaminophen level (at arrival and also at 4 hours after ingestion)
2. Use Nomogram
3. Consult Posion control
4. NAC (N-acetylcysteine), Admit
5. See Toxicology Section

54. Asthma - A 20 y/o with Wheezing, Cough and a History of Asthma
1. Wheezing, Cough, Hx Asthma, Dyspnea. When Severe: Retractions, Accessory muscle usage, difficulty speaking due to labored breathing. When even more Severe, Patient Not Moving Air and Lethargic/Fatigued
2. CXR and Treatments (Albuterol and Atrovent thrice, Steroids). If failing to respond to these, May add Magnesium sulfate, Epinephrine
3. If a Patient Does Not Improve (Status Asthmaticus), you need to admit them After Stabilization
4. Concerning findings in Asthma: Unable to Speak, Sit Forward, Use of Accessory Muscles/Retractions, Decreased Level of Consciousness, No Wheezing/Not Moving Air/Decreased Breath Sounds, Fatigue. These are All Signs of Impending Respiratory Failure
5. Questions to ask: History of Hospitalizations, History of Intubations, How Frequent are the Attacks, Current Asthma Medications. Frequency of the use of the Asthma Medications
6. Management: Beta Agonist (Albuterol) Nebs, Anticholinergic (Atrovent) Nebs, Steroids (Prednisone or Methylprednisolone). If still not working, Consider Magnesium, Epinephrine, Terbutaline. If still not working, Consider Bipap. Only If still not working and No other options, consider Intubation (Must Adjust Ventilator Settings because these Patients can be Susceptible to Pneumothorax etc. So if you must Intubate, Increase the Expiratory Time).

55. Diverticulitis - A 65 y/o with LLQ pain and diarrhea
1. LLQ Pain, Diarrhea
2. CT Abdomen/Pelvis
3. Management: IV Antibiotics (ie. Flagyl and Ciprofloxacin) and Definitely Admit if Intractable N/V/Pain/Complications such as Abscess, etc.

56. Epidural Abscess, Spinal Cord Compression, Cauda Equina Syndrome - A 40 y/o with Back pain and Diminished Rectal Tone
1. Neurological Deficit, Back Pain, Fever
2. Increased risk in IVDA, Immunocompromised Patients, Recent Spine Procedure
3. Needs STAT MRI
4. Loss of or Diminished Rectal Tone, Saddle Anesthesia, Weakness, Neurological Deficits, Back Pain, Leg Pain, Difficulty/Can't walk are all Possible findings, Possible Fever with the Former
5. IV Antibiotics, IV Steroids, STAT Neurosurgery Consultation for Surgical Decompression
6. Admit
7. If Not Promptly dealt with it can lead to Paralysis!

57. **Perforated Viscous (Perforated Duodenum, etc.) - A 30 y/o with Abdominal Pain, who is laying still on the stretcher due to pain. Exam shows Rebound Tenderness and Guarding**
    1. Chest X-ray may show Free Air under the Diaphragm
    2. Abdominal Exam likely with Rebound, Guarding (Patient is very uncomfortable)
    3. STAT Surgical Consultation and OR
    4. NPO, Give IV Antibiotics and initially on arrival send all labs including Pre-Op Labs. Stat Surgery Consult. Needs to go to the OR immediately

58. **Cholecystitis - A 40 y/o patient with RUQ pain, N/V and Fever**
    1. Inflammation of the wall of the Gallbladder
    2. RUQ pain, Fever, Nausea, Vomiting. Positive Murphy's Sign.
    3. Ultrasound RUQ (GB wall thickening, Pericholecystic Fluid, Sonographic Murphy's Sign, Distended GB, Gallstone), Stat Surgery Consult for Cholecystectomy, NPO, IV Antibiotics, IV Fluids

59. **Digoxin Toxicity - A 50 y/o patient with a history of Afib presents with Weakness**
    1. Nausea, Vomiting, Palpitations, Cardiac Arrest, Fatigue, Confusion, Visual Changes, Weakness, Altered Color Vision (ie Blue Green), Dizziness, Syncope, Arrhythmias
    2. Digitalis Blocks the Sodium Potassium ATPase Pump thereby causing Hyperkalemia
    3. DO **NOT** give Calcium for Hyperkalemia in a patient on Digoxin! It's **Contraindicated!**
    4. Immediately give Fab Fragments (Digibind or DigiFab) if Hyperkalemic and a Digoxin Toxicity Patient
    5. Reminder: Along with Potassium level send Magnesium level (supplement Magnesium if low)
    6. If Cardiac Arrest, follow ACLS guidelines but be sure to give DigFab/Digiband
    7. Bradycardia: May try ordinary measures (ie. atropine) but no guarantee it will work so always give Digoxin antibody fragments!
    8. Poison Control Consult

60. **Aspirin Overdose - A 41 y/o woman presents with Tinnitus**
    1. Send ASA level & Other Levels such as Acetaminophen Level, Alcohol Level, Toxicology screen, CBC, CMP, PT/PTT, Lactate, ABG, etc.
    2. Possible Symptoms and Findings Depending on Severity: Tinnitus, Nausea, Vomiting, Tachypnea, Metabolic Acidosis, Respiratory Alkalosis, AMS, Pulmonary Edema, Renal failure
    3. Consult Poison Control

4. Airway, Sodium Bicarbonate, Hemodialysis may be needed. ICU admit

61. Pyelonephritis - A 30 y/o woman with flank pain
   1. Kidney Infection, secondary to UTI ascending to the kidneys
   2. Send Labs, Cultures, Urinalysis, Urine culture
   3. Flank Pain (CVA Tenderness), Fever, Nausea, Vomiting, UTI symptoms (Dysuria, Increased Urinary Frequency are Possible), Positive UA. Treatment: IV Antibiotics, IVF's
   4. Admit Criteria Include: Pregnant, Persistent Pain/Nausea/Vomiting/Unable to Tolerate PO Antibiotics, Abnormal Labs, Elderly Patient, Failed Outpatient Treatment, Ill-appearing, Septic, Obstruction of urinary tract, Poor Compliance, Immunocompromised, Single Kidney, Uncertain of the Diagnosis
   5. If Patient meets Grounds for Discharge, you may give one IV dose of Antibiotics in the ER and then PO for home, but you must ensure Prompt Specialist follow up, Hydration, Antibiotics, etc.

Side Note: Imaging Tips:
1. An X-ray of Abdomen is used for SBO (May need a CT), Perforated Bowel Suspicion (Free air) and Foreign Bodies.
2. An Ultrasound is used for Gallbladder Etiologies (ie. Cholecystitis), Pregnancy, Ovaries (ie R/O Ovarian Torsion), Testicles (Testicular Torsion), Trauma US FAST exam.
3. A CT scan is helpful for many abdominal diagnoses: Appendicitis, Diverticulitis, Complications (Abscess), AAA Rupture, SBO, etc. Note: CT Abdomen/Pelvis Noncontrast is used for Kidney stones

62. Anaphylaxis - A 20 y/o man with Throat Swelling and Wheezing
   1. **Mnemonic for Treatment: RED MAN but remember ER (Epinephrine always first)**
      1. Ranitidine
      2. Epinephrine (this one is first…remember ER…Epinephrine before ranitidine)
      3. Diphenhydramine (Benadryl)
      4. Methylprednisolone/Prednisone
      5. Albuterol
      6. Normal Saline Bolus

63. Variceal Bleed - A 42 y/o Alcoholic with Hematemesis
   1. Hematemesis in Cirrhosis Patients
   2. A Form of Upper GI Bleeding (Other causes of UGIB: Variceal-Bleeding, PUD, Mallory Weiss Tear, etc.)
   3. Physical: Caput Medusae, etc.

4. CBC, CMP, PT/PTT, Type and Cross, Lipase, Alcohol level, EKG, CXR
5. IVF's, Octreotide, PPI, IV Antibiotics (ie. Ceftriaxone), Stat GI Consult for Emergent Endoscopy (Ligation, Sclerotherapy, etc). ICU Admit.

64. **Sepsis - A 60 y/o woman with Lethargy and Fever**
    1. Send Labs, Cultures, CBC, CMP, Lactate, Blood Cultures, Urinalysis, Urine Culture, Chest X-ray, CT Head? Lumbar Puncture? Any another study based on symptoms? Start IV Fluids early. Start Early IV Antibiotics. Central line? Pressors if fluids are not helping BP? Admit. Note: Consider Adrenal Crisis in patients BP not improving with the usual measures

65. **Carbon Monoxide Poisoning - A man, his dog and his family all have headache and weakness. The month is January and they live in a Cold Climate.**
    1. Headache, Seizure, Weakness, Confusion, Dizziness, Dysrhythmias, Dyspnea Ataxia, Nausea, Vomiting, Visual changes
    2. Dx: Carboxyhemoglobin Level
    3. Management: 100% Oxygen or Hyperbaric Oxygen in some Candidates
    4. Multiple Family Members, Pets may all be Symptomatic at the same time. More common in the Winter due to Space Heaters, etc.

66. **DVT - A 31 y/o with leg pain and swelling**
    1. Blood Clot in the Deep veins of the Lower Extremities (or Upper)
    2. If Untreated, concern is that it will travel to the lung vasculature and cause a Pulmonary embolism
    3. Leg pain, Leg swelling, Possible Redness
    4. Diagnosis is Ultrasound Doppler of veins (ie. of lower extremity deep veins)
    5. Management is Anticoagulation (ie. Lovenox), if No Contraindications
    6. If Untreated, can travel up and cause a blood clot in the Lungs (Pulmonary Embolism, which can be deadly if untreated). Risk factors: Prior DVT/PE, Family History of Thrombophilia, Immobilization, OCP use, Prolonged Travel, Recent Surgery, Obesity, Pregnancy, etc.

67. **Snake Bite**
    1. Always try to ask for descriptors of the snakes appearance (picture best)
    2. Send CBC, CMP, PT/PTT, Fibrinogen, Fibrinogen Split Products, UA, EKG, X-ray
    3. Call Poison control
    4. IVF's, Antivenin
    5. Crotalidae (ie Rattlesnakes): destroys local tissue around bite region. Can also lead to Ccoagulopathy and Neurological issues

6. Elapidae (ie. Coral snake) poison can cause symptoms hours later (Coral Snake with Red touching Yellow Pattern is Dangerous in the US). These snakes can case Neurological Symptoms and are Dangerous. Neurotoxicity. These patients need Antivenin and Admission.
7. Tetanus shot, Antivenin, Poison Control. Admit.

68. Cellulitis
1. Infection of Skin. Redness, Warmth, Swelling. Send Cultures. Give Antibiotics. Often times, also rule out a DVT with an Ultrasound Doppler in these scenarios.

69. Acute Narrow Angle Glaucoma - A 40 y/o with Abdominal Pain and Eye Pain
1. Headache, Eye Pain, Blurry Vision, Nausea, Vomiting, Abdominal Pain, Possibly see Halos around Lights
2. Physical Exam: Injected Conjunctiva, Shallow Anterior Chamber, Increased Intraocular pressure, A fixed, Mid-dilated pupil, Cloudy/Hazy Cornea
3. Slit lamp Exam, Tonopen shows elevated IOP
4. Emergent Ophthalmology Consultation and give the medications if not contraindicated (Topical Timolol, Topical Apraclonidine, Topical Pilocarpine, IV/PO Acetazolamide, IV Mannitol) - see eye section above

70. Gout, Pseudogout, Septic Arthritis, Gonococcal arthritis
1. A 30 y/o presents with pain in the big toe
2. A 20 y/o presents with a red, hot, swollen joint
3. Crystal Monoarthritis (Gout, Pseudogout)
4. Gout: Monosodium Crystals in Joint. Uric acid (Needle shaped and Negatively Birefringent). Arthrocentesis: Synovial fluid: Negative Gram Stain, Crystals with Monosodium Urate. Joint Pain (Very Painful), Warmth, Swollen, Erythematous. Can involve any joint but often times it's the Big Toe (Podagra). May see Tophi on affected area. Tx: NSAID.
5. Pseudogout: Calcium Pyrophosphate, Positively Birefringent Crystals in the Joints. Treatment: NSAID.
6. Gonococcal Arthritis: Rash, Fever, Joints involved. Neisseria Gonorrhea usually affects sexually active patients. The Joint (ie Knee or wrist or ankle or finger). The Patient can get Tenosynovitis, Polyarthritis and a Rash. You should send the Synovial Fluid from the Arthrocentesis for Gram Stain, Culture, Cell Count, etc. in these patients. You should also send Cultures of the Rectum, Throat and Genitals in these patients. Treatment: Antibiotics (ie. Ceftriaxone, Azithromycin).
7. Septic Arthritis (ie. Staph): Emergent. Joint pain, Swelling. Often preceded by Surgery, Trauma, Arthritis, etc. (Treatment: IV Antibiotics like Vancomycin + Ceftriaxone). Diagnosis: Arthrocentesis may or may not

show a positive gram stain. The WBC's will generally be greater than 50,000. Often Low Glucose. Needs STAT Orthopedic Consult

8. Diagnosis: Arthrocentesis (Send Synovial Fluid for Cell Count with Differential, Culture, Gram Stain, Crystals)
9. Treatments (See above)

71. **SCFE - A 13 y/o with Knee Pain and No trauma**
1. Often occurs in Obese Preteenage to Teenage Boys. Risk of Avascular Necrosis
2. The Femoral Head Epiphysis Slips
3. Can Present as Knee pain or Hip pain or Thigh pain or Groin pain
4. Often involves Both Femoral Heads so send X-rays of both Hips!
5. X-Ray of the Pelvis (views: AP, frog leg, lateral) is the Diagnosis
6. Management is Stat Orthopedic Consult, Patient Non-Weight Bearing, ORIF or Pinning

72. **Pneumonia - A patient with a Cough and a Fever**
1. CAP (Community acquired) vs HAP (Hospital acquired)
2. Fever, Chills, Cough, Lethargy, AMS possible
3. Management: IV Antibiotics (ie. CAP Tx: Azithromycin + Ceftriaxone)

73. **Cauda Equina Syndrome - A 45 y/o Patient with Back Pain and Urinary Retention**
1. Urinary Retention or Incontinence, Fecal Retention or Incontinence, Numbness/Weakness, Back Pain, Focal Deficits, Saddle Anesthesia, Poor Rectal Tone. Any of these possible.
2. STAT MRI needed
3. Stat Neurosurgery Consult Needed
4. May Start Steroids. If due to an Infectious cause (Epidural Abscess), Start Antibiotics

74. **Cardiac arrest**

1. *Scenario 1: A Patient suddenly collapses. He has No pulse. What steps would you follow at this point? (Follow the most uptodate ACLS guidelines). Imagine a scenario with Ventricular fibrillation or Pulseless Ventricular tachycardia (Hint: Defibrillation, CPR, Epinephrine...)*

2. *Scenario 2: A Patient suddenly collapses. There is a rhythm on the monitor but he has No pulse (PEA). What steps would you follow at this point? (Hint: Follow the most uptodate ACLS guidelines) (Hint: Look for and treat treat underlying cause:* **HAT Mnemonic,** *Epinephrine) -> See the following EKG!*

1. **HAT Mnemonic** *for Underlying Causes: Hypovolemia, Hypoxia, Hyperkalemia, Hypokalemia, Hypothermia, Hypoglycemia, Acidosis, Thrombosis (Myocardial Infarction, Pulmonary embolism), Toxins, Tension Pneumothorax, Cardiac Tamponade, Trauma*

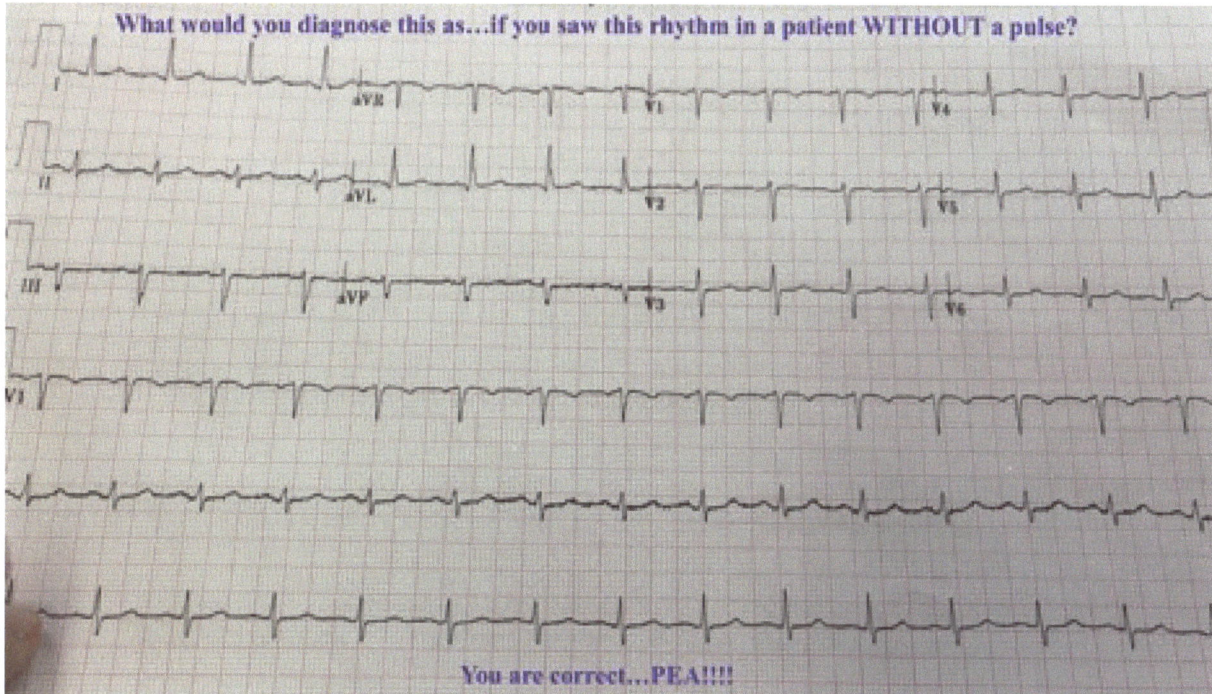

What would you diagnose this as...if you saw this rhythm in a patient WITHOUT a pulse?

You are correct...PEA!!!!

3. *Scenario 3: A Patient suddenly Collapses. He has No pulse. What steps would you follow at this point? Imagine a scenario with Asystole on the monitor (Hint: Follow the most uptodate ACLS guidelines)*

4. *Scenario 4: A patient suddenly collapses. He has a pulse. What steps would you follow at this point? (follow most uptodate ACLS guidelines). Imagine a scenario with a patient with Tachycardia with a Pulse*
   1. *Ventricular Tachycardia with a Pulse (If Stable: Amiodarone)*
   2. *Atrial fibrillation (Irregular) (Hint: Cardizem or Lopressor, if stable, for Rate Control. If Unstable: Cardioversion and "Unstable" means: Hypotensive, Chest Pain, AMS, Dyspnea)*
   3. *SVT : Narrow complex, Regular; Tachycardic. (Hint: Vagal Maneuver (ie. Valsalva), Adenosine if stable. Cardioversion if unstable)*
   4. *Atrial flutter: Presents with Sawtooth waves. What would you give/do?*

5. *Scenario 5: A patient suddenly collapses. He has a pulse. What steps would you follow at this point? Imagine a scenario with Bradycardia with a Pulse, with a syncopal episode. Hint: Follow the most uptodate ACLS Bradycardia guidelines*

75. **Sickle Cell Anemia: A Patient with Sickle Cell Anemia presents with Chest Pain and a Cough**
    1. Send Labs (CBC, CMP, Reticulocyte Count, Type and Cross, ABG, Cultures (Blood, Urine), Urinalysis, Chest X-ray, Possible CT Head (If CVA, AMS), Possible LP if Meningitis is a Concern). Give Oxygen, Give Fluids (if Acute Chest Syndrome, give carefully as they could get Pulmonary Edema). Give Pain medications. In cases of Infection or even Possible Infection, Give Antibiotics because Sickle Cell Patients are very prone to Infection! (Ask Allergies first). Note: EKG and CXR in all Chest Pain Patients.
    2. **Sickle Cell Crisis:** Bone Pain (ie Back Pain, Pain in Extremities). Is it like prior episodes or different?
    3. **Acute Chest Syndrome:** Dyspnea, Chest Pain, Fever, Cough, Possible Wheezing, New Infiltrate on CXR. Needs IV fluids, Oxygen, Pain medications, Antibiotics, Exchange Transfusion via Hematology-Oncology Specialty Stat Consult. Admit to ICU.
    4. **CVA (Stroke):** Stroke Symptoms. Needs Exchange Transfusion
    5. **Priapism:** Erect Penis. Needs IV Fluids, Pain Medications, Exchange Transfusion
    6. **Aplastic Crisis:** Serious Decline in Red Blood Cell Production often due to Infection. Low Hemoglobin Level, Low Reticulocytes. Severe Anemia (Concerning if Reticulocyte Count is <5. Low Reticulocyte Count is Bad). Often due to Parvovirus B19 Infection. May consider Transfusion.
    7. **Hemolytic Anemia:** Weakness, Anemia, Low Hemoglobin. Reticulocyte Count is Normal or High.
    8. **Osteomyelitis:** Joint with Tenderness/Redness/Swelling
    9. **Avascular Necrosis:** Consider with Hip pain in a Sickle cell patient
    10. **Splenic Infarction:** Due to lack/limitation of blood supply. In order to prevent infection, the patient needs Antibiotics (penicillin) and Immunization
    11. **Splenic Sequestration:** In children, presents with Splenomegaly (RBC's accumulate in the Spleen) and Anemia, Abdominal pain, Weakness. Treatment is Exchange Transfusion, Possible Splenectomy
    12. **Hand Foot Syndrome (Dactylitis):** Children usually under age 2. Swollen Hands and Feet, Painful.
    13. **Sepsis:** Needs Cultures drawn, Labs, Antibiotics.

76. CHF (Congestive Heart Failure) - A 65 y/o with Orthopnea and Dyspnea
1. Dyspnea, Pedal Edema, Dyspnea on Exertion, Orthopnea, Paroxysmal Nocturnal Dyspnea
2. Think of what the underlying precipitant may have been (ie. Myocardial Infarction, Aortic Stenosis, PE, Valvular issues, etc.)
3. Pro-BNP, CXR, Echocardiogram, Cardiology Consult
4. Nitroglycerin, Lasix and Management of the Underlying Cause

77. Ludwig's Angina - A 35 y/o with swelling of the submandibular region
1. Swollen Submandibular Region/Oral Soft Tissue Region, Due to Oral Infection
2. Jaw Pain, Dysphagia, Submandibular Area Swollen
3. Stat ENT Consult, Consider Early Airway Management, IV Antibiotics, ICU Admission

78. Henoch Schonlein Purpura (HSP)- A 7 y/o with Petechiae on the Lower Extremities and Buttocks
1. Purpura/Petechiae Rash on Legs, Buttocks
2. Rash, Abdominal Pain, Leg Arthralgia
3. Possible GI Bleeding, Renal Issues Possible
4. Diagnosis is Clinical and with Labs. Mostly Admit

79. COPD - A 70 y/o Smoker with Dyspnea
1. Dyspnea, Wheezing, Cough, Productive Cough, Smoking History
2. Oxygen, Albuterol/Atrovent, Steroids (Methylprednisolone or Prednisone), Antibiotics
3. CXR Portable
4. Consider Bipap if initial measures are Not working
5. Try to Avoid intubation in Asthma and COPD, if Possible unless unavoidable (adjust settings)

80. SVT
1. Narrow Complex, Regular with a Tachycardia.
2. Can be Symptomatic or Asymptomatic. May have Palpitations, May have Chest Pain, Syncope, Dizziness
3. Stable: Vagal Maneuvers (Valsalva Maneuver), Adenosine 6 mg Rapid IV Push with a Saline Flush afterwards if no response in 1 to 2 minutes, then you can give 12 mg Adenosine. If still No response, can give another 12 mg of Adenosine (this is all if the patient is stable. No cp/sob, etc)
4. Note if doses of Adenosine are Not working, Next you can try either a Beta Blocker or a Calcium Channel Blocker
5. Unstable (Chest Pain, Dyspnea, etc): Cardioversion Synchronized

81. Atrial Fibrillation
1. "Irregularly Irregular"
2. In a Hemodynamically Stable patient, **Rate control** of **Rapid** Atrial fibrillation is needed. This includes either a Beta blocker (ie Lopressor) or a Calcium channel blocker (ie Cardizem).
3. In Hemodynamically Unstable Patients, with Chest Pain, Dyspnea, etc. Cardioversion is needed.
4. Concerning Complication of Atrial fibrillation is a Stroke
5. Need to order Labs (including Cardiac Enzymes), EKG, CXR, Thyroid tests, Echocardiogram, Cardiology consult
6. In general, if a patient is stable, they consider anticoagulation prior to cardioversion, in those who are not on warfarin and in those in whom the atrial fibrillation has lasted over 48 hours.
7. Image: Atrial Fibrillation (Irregularly Irregular)

Atrial Fibrillation

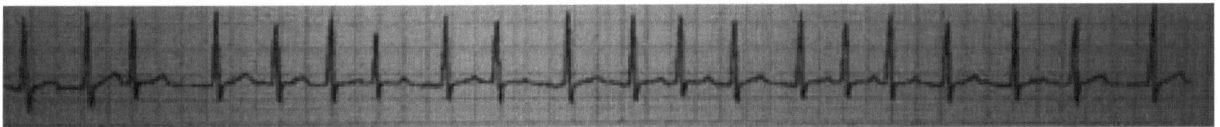

82. SJS (Steven Johnson Syndrome) - A Patient on Sulfa meds acquires a Target like Rash and Lesions on the Mouth
1. Rash (Target Lesions) and Mucosal Involvement (ie Eyes, Mouth)
2. Progression of Erythema Multiforme. SJS only: <10% TBSA. SJS/TEN involves 10 to 30% of Body surface area. Worse on the spectrum is Toxic Epidermal Necrolysis (involves >30% body surface area and skin sloughs off, desquamation). Often due to Medications (ie. Antibiotics, i.e. Sulfa Drugs). Management is to STOP the Medication that could be causing it. IV fluids, Replete Electrolytes. Consult the Burn Center. Admit.

83. Fournier's Gangrene - A 40 y/o man with Groin Pain
1. Dangerous Infection of the GU region at the level of the fascia. Physical exam may have Crepitus, Bullae, Erythema. More likely in Diabetics and Immunocompromised patients. Must have a High level of suspicion!
2. IVF's (NS), IV Antibiotics (Broad Spectrum), Stat Surgery Consult for Surgical Debridement

84. Hypoglycemia
1. Anxiety, AMS, Tachycardia. Precipitants: Medications (Insulin, Oral Hypoglycemics), Medical issues (Adrenal Crisis, Thyroid issues, etc), Alcohol, Temperature (Hypothermia). Reverse the Hypoglycemia with

Dextrose. In those with Sulfonylurea overdose, after dextrose, you can also give Octreotide. If the hypoglycemia is due to oral hypoglycemics (ie. sulfonylurea) or a moderate to long acting insulin, then the patient needs admission to prevent rebound hypoglycemia from going unnoticed/unmanaged.

85. **DKA (Diabetic Ketoacidosis) - A patient with Nausea, vomiting and a Blood Glucose of 400**
    1. **Mnemonic with DKA: PAINT CUP**
    2. Abdominal Pain, Weakness, Nausea/Vomiting, Polydipsia, Polyuria, AMS, Possible "Kussmaul's Breathing"
    3. Ketosis (High Ketones), Hyperglycemia (>250), Acidosis, Bicarbonate (<18)
    4. Precipitants: Noncompliance, Infection, MI, CVA...
    5. Please Check Labs Frequently and Reassess
    6. ABG
    7. Anion Gap (High)
    8. Antibiotics needed if underlying Infection
    9. Infection on the differential along with other possible triggers/etiologies
    10. Insulin
    11. ICU admit
    12. Normal Saline (2L NS and once glucose under 250, switch to D5 1/2 NS)
    13. Treat the underlying Cause, Talk to the patient and the family
    14. Chest X-ray
    15. Urinalysis and UHCG (pregnancy test)
    16. Possible Potassium Repletion Depending on Potassium Level. pH Low.
    17. Management: IVF's (NS), Regular Insulin IV. When Glucose reaches 250, Change IVF to D5 1/2 NS. Continue Insulin Drip until you Close the Anion Gap (Get Hourly FSG, ABG, Electrolyte Panel).

86. **Pyloric Stenosis - A Young Infant with Projectile Vomiting**
    1. Hypertrophy of the Pylorus musculature causing narrowing and thereby Nausea, Vomiting in a Young Infant
    2. "Projectile Vomiting"
    3. Infant is very Hungry, Dehydrated
    4. Metabolic Alkalosis
    5. Ultrasound = Diagnosis
    6. Treatment: Hydration, Surgery for Pylorotomy, Correction of Electrolytes

87. **Fever in a Neonate - A 3 week old infant with a Temperature of 102**
    1. Any Infant 28 days old or less needs a Full Septic Workup for a Fever
    2. CBC, CMP, Lactate, Blood Cultures, CT head (consider if focal neurological deficits, concern for mass, papilledema, etc.) and Lumbar puncture (CSF studies: Cell count with differential, Culture, Protein,

Glucose, Gram stain). Start IV Antibiotics after Blood Cultures and Start it Early if any concern for Meningitis.
3. Admit
4. Note: Always Obtain Informed Consent before any Procedure

88. **Boerhaave's - An Alcoholic who vomits and then suddenly gets Chest Pain**
   1. Full Thickness Perforation of the Esophagus
   2. Back pain, Chest pain, Neck pain Possible. Often before Forced Vomiting Episode.
   3. Dx: CT Chest if Stable. Unstable: Stat Surgery Consult for OR
   4. IV Lines x 2, IV Antibiotics, and STAT Surgery consult

89. **Testicular Torsion - a 15 y/o with Abdominal Pain, Nausea, Vomiting (Note: On your Testicular Exam: Horizontal Lie of the Testicle, Swollen and Tender, Absent Cremastueric Reflex)**
   1. Pain in the Testicle(s) or Abdomen. Nausea, Vomiting. Needs intervention immediately to save the testicle(s). Absent Cremasteric Reflex, Horizontal Lie, High Riding. Stat Urology Consultation. Ultrasound Doppler Testicles to Ensure blood flow. Also send the usual labs (CBC, CMP, PT/PTT, Type and Cross, Lactate, Urinalysis, etc.)
   2. Note: May Attempt manual reduction while awaiting admission to Urology OR. Note: Even if US read normal, testicles can torse and detorse, so keep it high in your differential.
   3. Key point: In a male with Abdominal pain, always do a chaperoned testicular examination! Torsion may present only with abdominal pain!
   4. Reminder: Torsion, if clinically suspected but not seen on ultrasound is still possible! It can torse and detorse, so when in doubt consult urology stat!
   5. Note: Epididymitis: UTI symptoms, Positive Urinalysis, Swollen, Tender Epididymis. Still get an Ultrasound in order to Ensure Good Testicular Flow. Give Antibiotics.

90. **Febrile Seizure - A 2 y/o with a fever and a single seizure lasting 10 seconds. She is back at baseline. Normal behavior. Otherwise, well appearing.**

   1. Simple Febrile Seizure: All of the below must be present in order to label it a simple febrile seizure
      1. Febrile Child (Temperature >/= to 100.4)
      2. Lasts Less than 15 minutes
      3. Child age: 6 months to 5 years old
      4. Within a 24 hour period, Only **One** seizure
      5. Well appearing child

6. Management: Identify cause of fever (Urinalysis, etc.) and ensure fever control management and discuss all symptoms/signs for immediate return with parents and importance of follow up, etc.
7. Note: Any criteria that doesn't fit all those listed above or in any child with meningeal signs, focal neurological deficits, ill appearance, medical history (prematurity, immunocompromised), age < 6 months old, afebrile, etc.) will need a more extensive workup for a seizure including labs, possible CT head, Lumbar puncture, etc.

91. Human Bite
1. A Human Bite needs Antibiotics, Tetanus shot, X-ray, Hand Surgeon and Extensive Irrigation, Splint in Neutral Position and Hand Surgeon/ Orthopedic Consult

92. Cat Bite, Dog Bite
1. **Mnemonic: TAXI FUR WOUND CHECK**
2. Tetanus immunization
3. Antibiotics (ie Augmentin)
4. X-ray Hand or region bitten
5. Irrigate wound
6. Follow Up appointment with Hand Specialist if discharging for wound check back to the ER or with PCP
7. Rabies discussion and prophylaxis per situation
8. Wound check in ER or with specialist
9. **A Human Bite Needs Antibiotics, Tetanus shot, X-ray, Hand Surgeon and Irrigation/Splint in Neutral Position and Hand Surgeon/ Orthopedic Consult**

93. Iron Overdose - A 22 y/o Overdoses on Iron tablets
1. GI (Abdominal Pain, Vomiting, Diarrhea, GI Bleeding). Suicidal?
2. CBC, CMP, PT/PTT, Type and Cross, Lactate, ABG, Serum Iron level, Cardiac Enzymes, Urinalysis, Call Poison Control
3. Stages: I: GI (Abdominal Pain, Vomiting, Diarrhea) II: Asymptomatic Often III: Lactic Acidosis, Shock, Coagulopathy, Liver or Kidney Failure, Cardiomyopathy. IV: Elevated LFT's
4. Treatment: Any Symptomatic Patients or those who are Unstable need IV Lines x 2, Cardiac Monitor, Oxygen, IVF's (If Hypotensive). Antiemetics if Nausea/Vomiting. Whole Bowel Irrigation with PEG. If Coagulopathy, consider FFP's and Vitamin K. Give Deferoxamine to Remove Iron from the blood in patients with Severe Poisoning (ie Toxic, Acidosis, etc). Needs ICU Admission
5. In anyone who is Asymptomatic for at least 6 to 8 hours of Observation and Never had any symptoms and Remains Asymptomatic, with Normal

Labs, Normal Vitals, Normal Appearance, Asymptomatic, No complaints, can consider sending home with close follow up.

6. However, anyone who had any symptoms at all at any time, should be Admitted for Observation, at the least, even if symptoms resolved, in order to ensure this is Not Stage II, where the patient presents Asymptomatic.

94. Epidural Hematoma - A 30 y/o with a Headache and AMS s/p Trauma
1. Bleed above the dura matter
2. Headache, AMS (may have periods where they fluctuate in and out of consciousness)
3. Young patients after a Trauma. Sudden Onset. Often due to Trauma of Middle Meningeal Artery
4. CT Head often shows a bleed shaped like a "Lens"
5. Neurosurgery Consult Stat
6. If very severe, consider evacuating immediately with a burr hole

95. Subdural Hematoma - A 60 y/o with AMS
1. Bleed below the dura matter
2. Headache, AMS
3. More often in Elderly Patients. Occurs over a longer duration
4. CT head
5. Neurosurgery Consult Stat

96. Kawasaki - A 4 y/o with 6 days of Fever, Conjunctivitis, an Erythematous Mouth/Hands/Feet and Lymphadenopathy
1. **Mnemonic: CHECK**
2. **CHECK Mnemonic: C**onjunctivitis, **C**ardiac complications, **C**ervical Lymphadenopathy, **C**racked Lips, **H**eart complications, **E**dematous hands/feet, **E**rythematous hands/feet, **E**rythematous Mouth/Lips, **K**awasaki
3. Can affect the Mucous Membranes, Heart, Skin, Lymph Nodes, Brain, Joints, etc.
4. Worst Complication: Coronary Artery Aneurysm, Sudden Cardiac Death
5. Fever for at least 5 days Must be Present, along with at least Four of any of the following: Conjunctivitis bilaterally, Lymphadenopathy in Cervical Region (Neck), Rash, Strawberry Tongue, Lips Cracked, Erythematous Mouth and Lips, Erythematous Hands/Feet, Edematous Hands/Feet, Desquamation
6. Treatment: Admit, IVIG, Aspirin, Cardiology Consultation
7. **CHECK Mnemonic: C**onjunctivitis, **C**ardiac Complications, **C**ervical Lymphadenopathy, **C**racked Lips, **H**eart Complications, **E**dematous Hands/Feet, **E**rythematous Hands/Feet, **E**rythematous Mouth/Lips, **K**awasaki

97. **Eclampsia - A postpartum woman who delivered a week ago presents with HTN and a Seizure**
    1. Always Suspect Eclampsia in a Seizing Pregnant Patient
    2. Always prepare for Impending Eclampsia in a Preeclampsia patient
    3. Preeclampsia = Proteinuria, Elevated BP. If Severe: Pulmonary Edema, Thrombocytopenia, Headache, Visual Changes, etc.
    4. Preeclampsia Treatment: Control BP with Hydrazine or Labetalol and Seizure Prophylaxis for Potential Impending Eclampsia with Magnesium
    5. Treatment = Magnesium to Prevent (and Treat) Seizures (Monitor for Hypermagnesemia Symptoms by Checking Reflexes (Decreased/Absent with Magnesium Toxicity). Magnesium Toxicity can lead to Respiratory Distress. OBGYN Consult Stat for Immediate Delivery of the Baby

98. **Croup - An 18 month old with a Barky cough at night**
    1. Viral illness (Often due to Parainfluenza). Barky cough, Stridor, Hoarseness, Preceding URI Symptoms. Febrile child. Often at Night.
    2. Corticosteroids (Dexamethasone), Nebulized Racemic Epinephrine
    3. ICU, ENT, Anesthesia if Impending Respiratory Arrest
    4. Reminder: Stridor, Retractions that don't resolve despite treatments or lethargy are all concerning and indicative of impending respiratory arrest

99. **Chest pain secondary to Cocaine use**
    1. **<u>Mnemonic: C-Milan</u>**
    2. **C** = Cocaine induced Chest Pain
    3. **M**orphine
    4. **L**orazepam (Benzodiazepine)
    5. **A**spirin
    6. **N**itroglycerin (**Contraindicated** if Inferior wall MI because it is a Preload Dependent State)
    7. What is **<u>Contraindicated</u>** in Cocaine induced Chest pain? Beta blockers are **Contraindicated**! (Never give this in cocaine induced chest pain because if beta blockade occurs then unblocked Alpha will run rampant!)
    8. Admit/Observation

100. **28 Days or Less with Fever:** Needs a Full Septic Workup and Admission! CBC, CMP, Blood Culture, Urinalysis, Urine Culture, Lumbar Puncture (CSF studies) as long as No Contraindications. Also can do CXR, RSV, Influenza. Give IV Antibiotics (Ampicillin, Cefotaxime or Gentamicin). Give Acyclovir if suspecting HSV. Must be Admitted.

101. **29 Days to 60 Days with Fever:** If Toxic/Ill appearing or High Risk, needs a Full Septic Workup and Admission. If Nontoxic/Well appearing, Full-term and Low risk do CBC, CMP, Blood Culture, Urinalysis, Urine Culture, Lumbar Puncture (CSF),

Ceftriaxone and Follow Up in 12 to 24 hrs. If Positive Blood Culture or No improvement or still with fever, Admit and give IV Antibiotics. What's Low Risk: Healthy, Well appearing, Full Term, Normal exam, Normal Labs, Normal Urine, Normal Stool, Normal LP results, Normal CXR, No Comorbidities, Normal Birth, Was Never on any antibiotics. Note: Anyone who is getting Antibiotics empirically needs an LP conducted first!

102. **60-90 Days with Fever:** If Toxic/Ill appearing or High Risk, then needs a Full Septic Workup and Admission. In those Unvaccinated, with Other illnesses, High Fever, also do a full workup. Send a Urinalysis and Urine Culture. Send Labs. Anyone with Respiratory Symptoms or High Fever or High WBC count Needs a Chest-Xray as well. Note: Anyone who is getting Antibiotics empirically needs an LP conducted first!

103. **Lisfranc Fracture:** A fracture of the Foot. There is a Fracture of the Base of the Second Metatarsal and there is a Gap between the First and Second Metatarsals. This needs Stat Orthopedic Consultation. An Unstable Lisfranc's injury Needs Orthopedic Surgical Repair

104. **Spontaneous Bacterial Peritonitis (SBP):** Abdominal Pain, Fever, Ascites Patient needs a Paracentesis (unless contraindicated). If neutrophils > or = 250 or Abdominal Pain/Fever in a patient with Ascites, then Needs Antibiotics (ie. Cefotaxime). Admit.

105. **Incarcerated Hernia:** Signs/Symptoms - Abdominal Pain, Nausea, Vomiting, Possible Fever. Irreducible (Incarcerated) or Strangulated (blood supply cut off) Please note: Emergent Surgical Consult needed if Incarcerated or Strangulated. Diagnosis: Physical Examination, CT scan Abdomen/Pelvis. Treatment/Management/Medications: NPO, IV Fluids, IV Antibiotics (ie. if Strangulated), Emergency Surgery Consult and Admission (if strangulated or incarcerated). Consultation/Disposition/Follow Up - Surgical Consult and Admission if Incarcerated or Strangulated Hernia or Persistent Pain/N/V. If Reducible Hernia and Asymptomatic, Surgical Follow Up

106. **Burn: To figure out how much of the body is burned, use the "Rule of 9's" rule:**
A Thermal Burn:

1. **First Degree Burn:** Painful Erythema of the Skin with solely Epidermal involvement
2. **Second Degree Burn:** Painful Erythema, Bullae, Blister with Epidermal and Dermal involvement
3. **Third Degree Burn:** Loss of Sensation over the Burn Site, White

"Rule of 9's": In an Adult, the Head, Neck is 9%, Front and Back of Chest is 18%, Front and Back of Abdomen is 18%, Each Upper Extremity is 9%, Each Lower Extremity is 18%, the Genitals are 1%

Any Singing of Facial Hair or any Swelling of the Face or any Carbonaceous Sputum or Any Signs of Shortness of Breath/Respiratory Distress/Stridor needs early intubation because these can all be indicative of inhalation injury. Intubate early because the Airway can get Edematous afterwards and it will be much harder to intubate. Must Consider Early Airway Management. Needs Tetanus shot, IV Fluids: 2 to 4 mL/kg of NS per % TBSA Burn: Give first half over first 8 hours and the rest over the next 16 hours, in a total 24 hour period. Consult Burn Center. Admit (if severe burn, moderate burn, any burn of the genitals, hands, feet, any joint or the pelvic region, any evidence of inhalation injury, Any partial thickness burn with >10% TBSA involved in adults, >5% TBSA involved in children, any third degree burn, lightning strike, electrical or chemical burn, elderly patient, pediatric patient, trauma, Circumferential burn, any comorbidities). These patients all need to be sent to a Burn Center immediately!

107. Myxedema Coma: Bradycardia, Hypotension, Hypothermia, Edema, Cold, Slow Reflexes, AMS, Hypoglycemia. Send Thyroid Tests (Free T4, TSH). Send Labs (CBC, CMP, etc). Do EKG. CT Head. Management is Airway first. Then, Levothyroxine and Steroids (ie. Hydrocortisone). You should give Steroids in the event that there is Adrenal Insufficiency concomitantly. Give IV Fluids. ICU Admission

108. Adrenal Crisis: Weakness. Hypoglycemia. Pigment Increased on Skin, Hyponatremia, Hyperkalemia (if Primary Adrenal Insufficiency). Nausea, Vomiting, Abdominal Pain, AMS. Send ACTH, Cortisol level and usual labs/ studies (CBC, CMP, FSG, EKG, etc). Patient needs Steroids! Treatment is Steroids! (Dexamethasone). IV Hydration. Admit to ICU!

109. ALTE (Apparent Life Threatening Event): Apnea in an infant. If infant turns blue or pale or has abnormal vital signs or syncope or becomes limp or the muscular tone changes in some way, then admit. ALTE can be representative of some very concerning findings (Infection/Sepsis/Meningitis/ Pneumonia, heart disease/arrhythmia, neurological issue (tumor, seizure, etc.), Trauma or Electrolyte imbalances. A thorough workup must be conducted. Labs (FSG, CBC, CMP), Blood Cultures, Urinalysis, Urine Culture, CT Head, Lumbar Puncture. EKG, CXR. Toxicologic studies. Cardiac Monitoring. Admit the Patient for Monitoring in order to ensure that there are no further episodes of apnea and also to attempt to find the underlying etiology of the ALTE.

A Few Helpful Key Points:

1. Any woman of childbearing age gets an HCG (qualitative, quantitative)
2. Everyone gets IV lines, O2 and Cardiac Monitor
3. Don't forget to ask for vital signs (all 6!)
4. Send Labs/studies! Do Appropriate Imaging studies!
5. Always think of the most detrimental diagnoses in all cases first (ie Tension Pneumothorax, Cardiac Tamponade, STEMI, Aortic Dissection, Ruptured AAA, Ectopic Pregnancy, Eclampsia, Ventricular Fibrillation, Ventricular Tachycardia, Pulmonary Embolism, CVA, TIA, Mesenteric Ischemia, Sepsis, Overdose, Symptomatic Bradycardia, Ovarian/Testicular Torsion, etc.)
6. If you don't know the dose to a medication, don't guess - state that you will look it up in an appropriate reference text
7. Draw your tables as soon as possible when entering the room (at times you may not be given the time, so memorize the table and practice a lot before the exam!)
8. There may be a case where you may not have a clear diagnosis, but it's the management that matters so know how to manage all scenarios and do so systematically!
9. There will be Single cases and Triple cases
10. Triple Cases: Always pick up where you left off with the prior patient (Ask all pertinent Questions listed in the box above and manage the patient appropriately and you will do well)
11. Triple Case Example...
    1. A 2 year old boy with Abdominal Pain
    2. A 56 year old woman with Weakness in her left leg
    3. A 40 year old presents after a Trauma (MVC) with Shortness of Breath

You will be presented the first patient. While working this patient up, the second one comes in and then the third one, comes in while you are working up the second one. Don't let this intimidate you. Memorize your table and follow the outlined table protocol drawn above for each patient. Practice Multiple scenarios together (Imagine the Labwork, EKG's, Chest X-rays, CT Head, Ultrasound (ie. US FAST), etc. that will be handed to you). Note that there are also E-oral Cases integrated into the Oral Boards in recent times. These will have the usual old-fashioned cases (pencil/paper) mixed with cases in which the examiner will also present you with video or audio, such as Imaging (CXR, Ultrasound, etc.), An Audio Call from EMS, etc. Look at the ABEM Website to Familiarize yourself with the Format of the Exam and Practice many cases and all that may be presented to you. Review all the cases presented to you in the Oral Boards Section and any other cases you may encounter.

Memorize and Follow the Table. Know your Diagnostic studies/Management Principles, Practice by yourself and with friends and you will do great. Good luck!

Sample Case: A 25 year old with Shortness of Breath after a penetrating trauma.

Vital Signs: BP 80/50, HR 120, O2 Sat 91%, RR 16, Temp 98.6

Follow the table above systematically for every case! (Ask for all 6 vital signs. Ask Family, EMS to stay, etc.)

Ask: **"What do I hear, see and smell?"** A man in respiratory distress who is AAO X 3

Primary Survey: (You will be expected to ask the findings you are looking for: ie. A: able to speak in full sentences? distress? B: tracheal deviation? breath sounds? C: Color of skin, Capillary Refill, CV auscultation, JVD
Airway: Patient is unable to speak in full sentences, breathing heavily
Breathing: Patient is in Respiratory Distress and has decreased breath sounds in the left lung and hyperresonance. You see Tracheal Deviation
Circulation: Pale, Distant Heart Sounds. JVD.

Interventions:
Oxygen by Nonrebreather mask. **Cardiac Monitor**. Place two large bore **IV Lines**. Ask the Nurse to **Send Labs** (CBC, CMP, PT/PTT, Type and Cross, Troponin, Lactate etc.) Give **IVF's**.
For the **Tension Pneumothorax**, This patient needs a **Stat Needle Decompression** followed afterwards by a **Chest Tube**.
This patient also needs a **Pericardiocentesis** (for **Cardiac Tamponade** if the patient is unstable in the ER). Stat Trauma, Surgical, Cardiothoracic Surgery Consult. Always **Reassess** after each procedure (be able to describe all procedures you conduct). The patient has improved. Now Collect a **History (HPI, PMH, Past Surgical History, Allergies, Social History, Family History)**.

Add additional Tests: EKG (showed Electrical Alterans), **Chest X-ray** after chest tube placement (CXR is normal if the Needle Decompression and Chest Tube were conducted in a timely fashion, prior to imaging). Do **Ultrasound FAST Exam**, Give **Pain medications** (note allergies!). **Echocardiogram** (at Bedside). Give Tetanus Shot.

Secondary Survey/Physical Exam: Head, Eyes, Ears, Nose, Throat, Lungs, Abdomen, GU, Back, Rectal, Extremities, Neurological, Skin.

Consults/Disposition: Cardiothoracic Surgery, Admit to the OR (Pericardial Window)

What are usually the **Critical (Mandatory) Measures** for the Oral Boards?

1. **Ask all of the information in the Table**
2. Diagnostic Testing where applicable (ie. X-ray, Ultrasound, CT). Ie. CVA? Bleed? Stat CT Head. Just Placed a Central Line or a Chest Tube? Needs CXR Post-Procedure! FSG, Labs, Tox Screen, Cardiac Enzymes, UA, Cultures, EKG, Echocardiogram, US FAST, X-rays
3. Medications (ie. Pain Medications, when the Patient is in Pain (Always Ask Allergies First!). Give Aspirin in a patient with a Negative CT Head getting admitted for a TIA or in a Cardiac Patient without Contraindications. BP Medication in a Patient with Aortic Dissection and High BP (ie. Beta Blocker and then Nitroprusside). In a Sepsis patient, IVF's, Blood Cultures and then IV Antibiotics all from early on. Stable Vtach: Amiodarone. Eclampsia Patient gets Magnesium and Needs Delivery. What would you give in a Thyroid Storm? Propranolol, PTU, Iodide (At least One hour after PTU, give Iodide), Steroid
4. Interventions: For instance: PCI for a STEMI. Operative Intervention (OR) for patient with a surgical issue (NPO, IVF's, Stat Surgery Consult, IV Antibiotics, etc).
5. Tetanus shot should be given for wounds, etc.
6. Look at Labs and Correct as needed. For instance: How would you Treat Hyperkalemia? Hypoglycemia?
7. Manage each individual situation as well. For example, Cooling if Hyperthermic. Give the appropriate Antidote for Toxicology Patients.
8. Appropriate Consult: i.e. Neurology for CVA/TIA. Cardiology/Cath Lab for STEMI. Surgery for Surgical issue (ie. Appendicitis), OBGYN (ie. for Ovarian Torsion). Eclampsia needs stat OB, Magnesium, Delivery. Get the Urologist for Testicular Torsion, Get GI for a Variceal Bleed, etc.
9. Trauma patients need a Stat Trauma consult and a Full Evaluation (CBC, CMP, T&C, PRBC's, X-rays (Chest, Pelvis), C-S Immobilization, US FAST. If stable, Possible CT scan vs. If Unstable: Stat Surgery Consult for OR, etc).
10. Isolation as needed (ie. TB patients, Meningitis patients).
11. HCG test must be sent in women! Always Remember the Pregnancy Test!
12. Admit the Patients who need to be Admitted to the appropriate level of care (ie. ICU)
13. Perform Timely and Appropriate Procedures and be able to Describe them. For instance: Needle Decompression, Chest Tube for Tension Pneumothorax. Lumbar Puncture for Meningitis. Ventricular Fibrillation and Pulseless Ventricular Tachycardia need Defibrillation.
14. Reassess the Patient after Every Intervention to ensure they are Improving
15. The Diagnostic/Treatment Modality for each Pathology (For instance: Intussusception will need an Ultrasound for Diagnosis. It needs a Surgery Consult. IR Consult. Air Enema is often both Diagnostic and the Treatment Modality. If this doesn't work, Surgical Management is the Next Step).

Section IV: Rapid Review! Quick Questions & Answers and A Quick Review of Major Concepts to Know

1. A Man has RUQ pain, Fever, Nausea, Vomiting, Positive Murphy's sign. Next step? Labs, RUQ Ultrasound, IVF's. His RUQ US shows Cholecystitis. Next step? IV Antibiotics and Stat Surgery Consult for a Cholecystectomy

2. EMTALA: You must provide every patient who walks through the ER with a Medical Screening Examination to ensure that if there is a Medical Emergency, you will immediately Intervene in order to Help Stabilize the Patient. Only if the services are unavailable at your hospital, to stabilize the patient, can you transfer the patient.

3. A Patient has a Retrobulbar Hematoma (Proptosis, etc). What do you do next? Lateral Canthotomy and Ophthalmology Consult Stat.

4. You Diagnose Fournier's Gangrene in a Patient. What's the Next Step? Stat Surgery Consult for Surgical Debridement and IV Antibiotics, IV Fluids.

5. A Patient with Atrial fibrillation tells you she has Severe Pain. On Physical Examination, Abdomen is Nontender. Lactate is elevated. What do you think this might be? Mesenteric Ischemia. What do you do next? Stat Consult to Surgeon, IR. IVF's, IV Antibiotics.

6. A Patient has a Cloudy Cornea, a Mid-Dilated Pupil that doesn't react. What could this be and What is Diagnostic? Acute Narrow Angle Glaucoma (Tonopen shows Elevated IOP). What do you do next? Stat Ophthalmology Consult and Give Medications (ie. Topical Timolol, Topical Apraclonidine. Topical Pilocarpine. IV Acetazolamide. IV Mannitol).

7. A Patient has Fever, Neurological Symptoms, Thrombocytopenia, Renal Failure and Anemia. What do you think they have and What is the Management?
TTP and Plasmapheresis. TTP Mnemonic is No FART!

8. A Person has a Swollen, Tender Joint. What should you do? Arthrocentesis. What's the major concern that you are trying to rule out? Septic Arthritis. What's the treatment if this is what the results demonstrate? IV Antibiotics, Stat Orthopedic Consult. Admit. What Physical Exam Finding might you find in Septic Arthritis? Pain on Passive Motion.

9. If the results of an Arthrocentesis showed Positively Birefringent Calcium Pyrophosphate Crystals, what would you think? Pseudogout

10. If the results of an Arthrocentesis showed Negatively Birefringent Urate Crystals, what would you think? Gout

11. If a woman in her late teens to early 20's started to have Multi Systemic Symptoms, in addition to a Fever and a Rash and she is on her Menstrual Period and has a Tampon in at present, what should you consider? Toxic Shock Syndrome. What is the Management? IVF's, IV Antibiotics, Remove the Tampon and Admit

12. Name Two Scenarios (One involving the Eyes and one involving the Ears that are predisposed to Pseudomonas infections and where you have to cater the antibiotics to cover for pseudomonas). A Contact Lens User with a Corneal Ulcer. A Person who swims, with Otitis Externa (Swimmer's Ear)

13. How is a Jellyfish Sting Managed Differently from a Stingray one?
Jellyfish: Put Vinegar on the Sting Site and for a Stingray, put Hot Water over the lesion

14. What's the Management of a Bite from a Coral Snake that has Red Bands next to Yellow Bands? Antivenin! They are often Neurotoxic, so even if the patient initially manifests as asymptomatic or with minimal symptoms, Always Admit for Monitoring!

15. What is the Treatment for Anaphylaxis? Mnemonic: RED MAN but ER first (Epinephrine First)! Epinephrine, Ranitidine, Diphenhydramine (Benadryl), Methylprednisolone, Albuterol, Normal Saline

16. What shouldn't you give in a patient with an Inferior wall MI, Right ventricular Infarction? They are Preload Dependent, so give them IV Fluids, but **Avoid** giving them Nitroglycerin, Diuretics, and Morphine (These are **Contraindicated!)**

17. Which STEMI has ST Depressions in leads V1, V2? Posterior wall MI

18. What is the Diagnosis for Testicular Torsion? Ultrasound of the Testicles with Doppler Flow. Management? Stat Urology Consult for OR. Always keep Torsion on your Differential if a patient has Abdominal Pain or Testicular Pain or Nausea/ Vomiting

19. A Man has Back Pain, Chest Pain and Numbness in his Lower Extremity. There is a Pulse Deficit on Exam and an Aortic Regurgitation Murmur. His Vitals show that he is Moderately Hypertensive. What is the Diagnosis? What is the Ideal Diagnostic Testing in Stable Patients? What is the Management? Aortic Dissection. CT Chest/ Abdomen. Stat Vascular Surgery Consult for OR repair and if HTN present, Management needed with a Beta blocker and Nitroprusside. The Beta blocker is given first in order to avoid reflex tachycardia!

20. On an EKG, you see some Deep Inverted Symmetrical T waves in leads V1, V2. What is this and What should you do and why? Wellen's syndrome. Send to the Cath Lab because these patients have Severe LAD Stenosis!

21. A 15 year old boy passed out. He has a Positive Family History of Early Cardiac Death. What should you do with this patient after the usual workup? Cardiology, Echocardiogram, Admit for possible Hypertrophic Cardiomyopathy

22. A Patient has PND, Orthopnea, DOE, Bilateral Pedal Edema. What is this? What is the General Initial Management of this Condition? CHF. Nitroglycerin, Lasix. Oxygen. Search for the Precipitating Cause that led to the CHF. Pro-BNP, Echocardiogram are the Diagnostic Modalities. If still trouble breathing despite Oxygen and the Patient is Alert, try Bipap.

23. A Smoker Presents with Wheezing and a Cough. CXR is Hyperinflated. What is this likely to be? What is the Initial Management when they come in? COPD. Oxygen, Albuterol nebs, Atrovent nebs, Steroids, Antibiotics, Admit.

24. A Patient presents with Wheezing and has a History of Asthma. What Medications should you give? Albuterol, Atrovent, Steroids. If these are not working, what are other medications to consider? Magnesium, Epinephrine, Terbutaline

25. A Patient presents with Nausea, Vomiting. He overdosed on Digoxin. What is the Main item that must be give? Digoxin antibody fragments (Digiband)

26. What is **Contraindicated** in Digoxin patients? Calcium!

27. A Renal Patient is shown to have Wide QRS Complexes on EKG and a Potassium of 7.8. What should you give the patient? Calcium, Insulin, Glucose, Albuterol, Sodium Bicarbonate, Kayexalate, Dialysis

28. In Symptomatic Patients with Third Degree Heart Block, What needs to be Done? Pacing!

29. An Elderly Man Presents with Abdominal Pain and Syncope. His vitals show Borderline Hypotension. What Test should be done? Ultrasound Abdomen. (If Stable, CT Abdomen/Pelvis). The Ultrasound shows that he has a Large AAA that is 6.5 cm in size. What is the Next Step? Stat Surgery Consult to go to the OR for Lap. Give Fluids, PRBC's.

30. A Patient has a Rhythm on the Monitor but No Palpable Pulse. What does this mean? The patient is in PEA! What should you do? Follow the latest ACLS guidelines (CPR, Epinephrine, Search for underlying causes: Mnemonic is HAT -

Hypothermia, Hypovolemia, Hypoxia, Hypokalemia, Hyperkalemia, Hypoglycemia, Acidosis, Trauma, Thrombosis (MI, PE), Toxins, Tamponade (Cardiac), Tension Pneumothorax

31. What does the EKG look like in an Inferior wall MI? ST elevations in at least two contiguous leads of II, III, avF and ST depressions in I, avL. You should get the Right sided Leads (V3R, V4R showing an ST Elevation) to Look for a Right Ventricular Infarction.

32. If a Patient's X-ray comes back Normal but they have Tenderness over the Scaphoid Bone (Snuffbox Tenderness), What do you do? Thumb Spica Splint and Prompt Orthopedic Follow Up because Scaphoid Fractures may not show on Initial X-rays for days to weeks

33. What is the Diagnostic Test and Management for Appendicitis? CT Abdomen/ Pelvis (RLQ US in children if possible) and Stat Surgery Consult for OR, NPO, IV Antibiotics and Admit

34. A Woman presents with Vaginal Spotting. What are the Next Steps? Get labs (CBC, CMP, PT/PTT, Type and Screen), Urinalysis, HCG Qualitative, Quantitative. HCG is positive. What's the Next Step? Transvaginal Ultrasound. Results show a Possible Ectopic Pregnancy and No IUP. Patient is stable. What's next? Stat OBGYN Consult to decide if the patient should be Managed with Methotrexate (Stable and meets all the criteria for Methotrexate Administration) or if the patient is Unstable or Doesn't meet all of the criteria for Methotrexate administration, then the patient needs to go to the OR for a Lap.

35. What are a few concerning things you should worry about in a patient with Back Pain and Neurological deficits? Spinal Cord Compression, Aortic dissection.

36. If a Patient has Back Pain, Leg Pain, Saddle Anesthesia and a Diminished Rectal Tone, What are you worried about and What is the Management? Cauda Equina Syndrome. Needs Stat MRI and a Stat Neurosurgery Consult. Start Steroids to Lessen Edema. If an Infection is the Underlying Etiology (ie Epidural Abscess), Give IV Antibiotics as well.

37. A Patient has No breath Sounds Unilaterally, JVD and Tracheal Deviation. What is this and What's the Treatment? Tension Pneumothorax. Needs Needle Decompression and a Chest Tube

38. What is the Treatment for Gas Gangrene? IV Antibiotics, IV Fluids and Surgical Debridement (Stat Surgical Consult)

39. A Patient has Muffled Heart Sounds, JVD and Hypotension. What is this and What's the Treatment? Cardiac Tamponade. Pericardiocentesis.

40. A Child has a Bark-like Cough and URI symptoms. What do you think this is and What is the Management? Croup. Give Dexamethasone, Nebulized Racemic Epinephrine

41. What do you do if your Patient has Rebound, Guarding and Free Air under the Diaphragm? What is this? Perforated Viscous. Stat Surgery Consult, IV Antibiotics, IVF's

42. What is the Management for Torsades? Defibrillation, Magnesium

43. What is the Management for Ventricular Fibrillation or Pulseless Vtach? Defibrillation

44. What is the Management for SVT (Stable)? Valsalva initially and if this doesn't work, Adenosine. If Unstable: Cardioversion

45. What is the Management for Atrial Fibrillation (Unstable)? Cardioversion
If Stable: Rate Control with Beta Blocker or Calcium Channel Blocker

46. A Man has Abdominal pain, Constipation, Nausea, Vomiting and a History of Many Abdominal Surgeries. What do you think? Small Bowel Obstruction (SBO). Diagnosis: Xray Abdomen Flat and Erect may show Air-fluid levels. CT Abdomen/ Pelvis shows Complete SBO. What is the Management? NPO, IVF's, NG tube, Stat Surgery consult, Admit. What are the Two Main Causes of SBO? Adhesions (from prior surgeries) and Hernias.

47. What is the Management in a Patient who is under 28 days old with a Temperature of 101? Needs a Full Septic Workup! (Labs, Blood Culture, Urinalysis, Urine Culture, Chest X-ray, (Possible CT Brain if concerned for a Mass lesion), Lumbar puncture with CSF studies, IV Antibiotics after Cultures and Admit). Remember in these patients you need Ampicillin for Listeria coverage. Will also need to use Cefotaxime as One of the Antibiotics (**Not** ceftriaxone!)

48. A patient presents after a TCA overdose. What is the Management? Sodium Bicarbonate

49. In a patient who has a Subarachnoid Hemorrhage on CT, what symptoms might you expect and What is the Management? Nausea, Vomiting, Headache, Neck Stiffness, Photophobia. Neurosurgery consult. Nimodipine to prevent vasospasm

50. In a Patient with Meningitis What Symptoms do you expect and What is the Management? Nausea, Vomiting, Fever, Chills, Headache, Neck Stiffness, Photophobia. Labs and cultures, Needs CT brain if any concern for a Mass. After this, needs an LP, if not contraindicated with CSF studies (Cell Count with Differential, Gram Stain, Glucose, Protein and any additional studies). After sending Blood Cultures, Give Steroids and IV Antibiotics.

51. What do you do in a Patient with Cirrhosis, Ascites, Abdominal Pain, Fever? Paracentesis, IV Antibiotics, Admit

52. What is seen in Cholangitis? Fever, Jaundice, RUQ pain. When Severe, may also have Altered mental status and Hypotension. What is the Management? IV Antibiotics, ERCP, Stat Surgery and GI Consults. Admit.

53. A Pregnant Patient has HTN and a Seizure. What is your concern? What is the Management? Eclampsia. For Eclampsia, Give Magnesium sulfate and the Patient Needs Immediate Delivery! Additional HTN treatment is Labetalol or Hydralazine.

54. What is Contraindicated in Placenta Previa or Possible/Suspected Placenta Previa? A Pelvic exam is **Contraindicated!** How do you make the Diagnosis? An Abdominal Ultrasound.

55. What is the Diagnosis of a Kidney Stone? Noncontrast CT Abdomen/Pelvis. Management is IV Fluids and Medications for Pain, Urology

56. What is the Best Treatment for Acute Mountain Sickness, HACE and HAPE? Descent

57. What is one of the diagnoses you should consider in a child with a Knee pain or Thigh pain? Consider SCFE. Do Bilateral Hip X-rays. Management is Stat Orthopedic Consult for ORIF. Don't let the Patient Bear Weight.

58. What do you suspect in a Patient on Oral Contraceptives who flew into NY from Australia two weeks ago, who presents with Chest pain and Dyspnea? Pulmonary Embolism. Management is Anticoagulation. Risk factors for PE are Prolonged Immobilization (Long Travel, Recent Surgeries), Malignancy, OCP use, Prior History of DVT or PE, Family History of Thrombophilias, Obesity, Pregnancy.

59. Beta Blocker Overdose can present with Hypotension, Bradycardia, Hypoglycemia. Give Glucagon

60. Calcium Channel Blocker Overdose can present with Hypotension, Bradycardia, Hyperglycemia. Give Insulin.

61. Ruptured Globe: Needs Stat Ophthalmology Consult for Operative Repair. Shield the Eye. Give Tetanus shot and Antibiotics. What is **Contraindicated?**
Never use a tonopen in these patients! This is Contraindicated!

62. An Alcoholic presents with Hematemesis. What do you think is going on? Esophageal Varices. IV, O2, Monitor, IVF's, PRBC's if needed, Antibiotics, Octreotide, Stat GI consult because Stat Endoscopy is needed.

63. Pheochromocytoma: Presents with HTN, Tachycardia, Sweating, Headache, Palpitations, Anxiety. Due to Excessive Catecholamine Release. Management is Alpha Blocker, Phenoxybenzamine and Surgical intervention.

64. What do you suspect in a patient with a Fever and a Murmur? Endocarditis. What is the Diagnosis? Echocardiogram and Blood Cultures. What is the Management? IV Antibiotics

65. What are Transplant Patients prone to? Infection, Rejection, Immunosuppressant Toxicity

66. What do you do in a Patient with Epigastric pain Radiating to the Back? There are many differentials, but one to consider is Pancreatitis. What is one of the blood tests you should order that will likely be abnormal? Lipase. What is the Management? IVF's and Admit. If any Complications are a concern, do CT scan and proceed from there.

67. A Patient drank lots of Alcohol and then Profusely Vomits. He then has Chest pain, Neck pain, Back pain. What do you think is going on? How do you manage it? Boerhaave's Syndrome. Stat Surgery Consult for Surgical Repair, IV Antibiotics.

68. What should you do for a TIA? CT Head (if No bleed, give Aspirin). Consult Neurology. Admit to Neurology for Echocardiogram, Carotid Doppler and MRI. TIA patients have an Increased Risk of having a Stroke in the next 48 hours.

69. What do you suspect in a patient with Chorea, Nodules on the Skin, Rash (Erythema Marginatum), Arthritis, Endocarditis? Rheumatic Fever. What is the Management? Antibiotics.

70. What is the Management for Fournier Gangrene? IV Antibiotics and Stat Surgical Debridement

71. TEN is at the End of the Spectrum of EM, SJS, TEN. TEN causes a + Nikolsky sign and is due to medications like sulfa drugs. The first step is to Stop the Medication causing the issue. Patient needs IVF's and Admission to the Burn Unit.

72. Henoch Schonlein Purpura (HSP): Rash on the Lower Extremities/Buttocks. May also have a Renal issue, Abdominal pain, Joint pain.

73. What do you give a Stable Patient with a Pulse who has Ventricular Tachycardia? Amiodarone

74. What are signs of a Basilar Skull Fracture? CSF Otorrhea, CSF Rhinorrhea, Racoon's eyes, Hemotympanum, Battle sign

75. If you have a Patient with Visual Loss and No pain and the exam shows a Pale Retina and a Very Red Macula, what would you call it? CRAO. How is this managed? Consult Ophthalmology and Massage the globe intermittently. Why? To Dislodge the Clot. Who is Predisposed to this? Cardiac Patients, Patients with Atrial Fibrillation

76. In a patient with Pain in the Temporal region, who is Elderly what do you Suspect? Temporal Arteritis. What do you do? ESR is high, Ophthalmology Consult Stat to Prevent your patient from going Blind and Immediately give Steroids when you suspect Temporal Arteritis

77. What is the Main Management for DIC? Treat the underlying cause.

78. What do you see in a Patient with Adrenal Crisis? Hypoglycemia, Hypotension, No response to IV fluids. What should you give them? Steroids. ICU admit.

79. Why should you do a Urinalysis on a Pregnant woman? They can have Asymptomatic Bacteriuria and this Needs Treatment (ie. Nitrofurantoin = Macrobid)

80. In a Pediatric Patient (Infant) who is Crying and Legs are "drawing upward", what do you suspect? Intussusception. How does it present? Abdominal pain, Nausea, Vomiting, "Draws Legs Upward" towards abdomen, due to pain. What is the Diagnosis and Management? The Diagnosis is Ultrasound in Children and CT scan in Adults. Stat Surgical Consult. Management in Children and at times the Diagnosis is a Contrast Enema (Air Enema). If there is Perforation or if the Air Enema doesn't work, the patient needs Stat Surgery (Laparotomy). In Adults the Management is Surgical.

81. What is very Important to do in a patient with Kawasaki disease? Consult Cardiology for Echocardiogram for Coronary aneurysms. Give IVIG, Aspirin. How does it present? Mnemonic: CHECK: Conjunctivitis, Cardiac complications, Cervical

Lymphadenopathy, **C**racked Lips, **H**eart complications, **E**dematous hands/feet, **E**rythematous hands/feet, **E**rythematous Mouth/Lips, **K**awasaki

82. What do you see on the X-ray for Epiglottitis, if the Patient is Stable enough to have one done? Thumbprint sign. What should you do in these patients? Airway Management is a Priority. ENT consult. IV Antibiotics. Let the patient stay in a Comfortable position. ICU Admit.

83. A Patient with a Cold/Pulseless Foot needs what? Immediate Vascular Surgery Consult for Stat OR

84. In a Patient with Delirium Tremens, due to Alcohol Withdrawal, Hemodynamically Unstable vitals present (ie. Hypertension, Tachycardia). Can be Anxious or have a Tremor. May have a Seizure. Needs Lorazepam (Benzodiazepine) and ICU Admission.

85. Anticholinergic Toxidrome: AMS, Urinary Retention, HTN, Tachycardia, Dry, Hyperthermia

86. What is the Management of Cerebral Venous Thrombosis? Anticoagulation

87. What is the Management for Methemoglobinemia? Methylene Blue

88. Anterior or Posterior Packing Needs Antibiotics! Posterior Nasal Packing Needs Admission because many complications can result.

89. What is your Concern in an Elderly Diabetic with Ear Pain? Malignant Otitis Externa

90. What are the Symptoms of Iron Poisoning and the Treatment? It affects the CNS, Kidneys, GI system, Heart. Management is Whole Bowel Irrigation with Polyethylene Glycol and also Deferoxamine for a Severe Overdose

91. What is the Management for PCP pneumonia? Trimethoprim-Sulfamethoxazole and Steroids (Give Steroids if the A-a gradient is > 35 or PaCO2 is <70)

92. Corneal Ulcer: Needs Stat Ophthalmology Consult, Antibiotics

93. SVC Syndrome: In Patients with Malignancy, can have Facial Swelling, Arm Swelling, Dyspnea, Cough, Dysphagia

94. In a patient with Malaise, Sore Throat and a Positive Monospot Test, What is the Diagnosis and What is the Management? Infectious Mononucleosis. Supportive care

and Advise against Contact Sports since these patients are at Increased Risk of Splenic Rupture.

95. What is the Management of Cavernous Sinus Thrombosis? IV Antibiotics

96. Mallet Finger: Occurs due to Hyperflexion of the Distal Finger (DIP). Treatment is to Splint the DIP in Extension for 2 months

97. High Pressure Injection Injury: Needs Stat Hand Surgery/Orthopedic Consult for Debridement and IV Antibiotics and Admission

98. WPW: Slurred upstroke of QRS is present and known as a Delta wave. If the patient is stable, consider Procainamide in Stable Patients. WPW is Due to an Accessory Pathway.

99. There is Blood at the Urethral Meatus. What are you Concerned About? What Test should be done to Confirm? What should you Avoid prior to Testing? Urethral Injury. Avoid Foley. Diagnosis is a Retrograde Urethrogram.

100. Compartment Syndrome: Need to Measure Compartment Pressure. Needs Stat Fasciotomy. Patient presents with some of the following: Pain, Paresthesia, Pallor, Cool skin/Cold skin, Pulselessness. These can happen due to many risk factors, such as a Fracture/Cast. Elevated Compartment Pressure. Needs Stat Orthopedic Consult. Fasciotomy.

101. A patient travels to the Southeast part of the United States and when he returns, with his family, he gets myalgias, a headache and a petechial rash that begins on the wrists and ankles and then travels to the trunk. What is this classic description and what is the management? Rocky Mountain Spotted Fever and the Treatment is generally Doxycycline. What lab findings can possibly be found in RMSF? Hyponatremia, Thrombocytopenia. What should you always ensure is not going on in a patient with Headache, Fever, Nausea, Vomiting, and a Petechial Rash? Meningitis!

102. What is the Management of an Auricular Hematoma? It needs immediate I & D and Packing because otherwise leads to Major Deformity of the Ear due to Lack of Blood Flow.

103. A Patient has Abdominal pain and Hematochezia. He had a Cardiac Procedure in the past but he cannot recall what it was. What is your concern and how do you Manage it? Aortoenteric Fistula. Needs Stat Surgical Consult for Repair.

104. A Patient has been taking an SSRI and some other medication known to cause Serotonin Syndrome when both combined. What is the Management for this? Cyproheptadine. How can Serotonin Syndrome present? HTN, Tachycardia, AMS, Fever, Reflexes Increased, Clonus, Tremor.

105. Neuroleptic Malignant Syndrome: HTN, Tachycardia, AMS, Rigidity, Fever, Reflexes Decreased etc. Management is Supportive and Dantrolene

106. How do you treat PID? Ceftriaxone + Azithromycin/Doxycycline + Metronidazole

107. What can a Heat Stroke present with? What is the Main Principle of Management? Temperature very high (>104), Headache, Seizure, Syncope, Confusion. Management is Immediate Cooling, Cool IVF's

108. A Basketball Player's Finger gets latched onto another players shirt. He is unable to flex the DIP of that digit. What is this and what does he need? Jersey finger. Needs Orthopedic for Surgery.

109. Cyanide poisoning Treatment: Amyl Nitrite, Sodium Nitrite, Sodium Thiosulfate. How does Cyanide Poisoning Present? AMS, Hypotension, Tachycardia, Nausea, Vomiting, Dyspnea, Dysrhythmias, Headache, Seizure

110. A Right Handed Man Presents with Swelling, Erythema and a Small Laceration to his Right Knuckle area. He says that he fell. What should you suspect and what should you do? This could be secondary to punching someone's teeth (Clenched Fist Injury = Fight Bite). It can lead to a Serious Infection. Many patients don't like to admit this due to embarrassment. Always err on the side of caution because it can lead to major deformities. He needs IV Antibiotics, Stat Hand Surgeon/Orthopedic Consult, Irrigate the wound, Tetanus Shot, X-ray, and Admission.

111. Flexor Tenosynovitis: Swollen Digit, Passive Extension leads to Pain, Holds Digit Slightly Flexed, Pain along the Flexor Tendon Sheath when touched. Needs IV Antibiotics immediately and Stat Hand Surgeon/Orthopedic Consult for Operative Repair.

112. What is a Hyphema? How do you Manage a Hyphema? Aqueous Humor of the Anterior Chamber fills with Blood. It can cause pain in the eye and on eye exam you can clearly see blood accumulation. It needs a Stat Ophthalmology Consult. Additionally, Shield the eye and keep the Patient Sitting Upright. No strenuous activity. Often due to trauma, sickle cell anemia, or a bleeding disorder. The Patient should be Admitted.

113. A Woman comes in with Abdominal pain and Vaginal discharge. Her pregnancy test is Negative. On exam, you note that there is CMT, Adnexal Tenderness and a Palpable Adnexal Mass. She states that she recently had an infection down there and was treated with some medications she cannot recall the name of. She had a recent pelvic surgical procedure. What is your next step? What is the management of the condition you find? The next step is a Transvaginal Ultrasound. It shows a Tubo-Ovarian Abscess. Patient needs IV Antibiotics and Needs to be Admitted. Stat Consult to OBGYN service.

114. A Patient Sustained a Trauma. During your Physical Exam, you notice that the Pelvis is Unstable. What should you immediately do for the Pelvis at that point? Place a Pelvic Binder. Note: Rule out Hemorrhage in the Chest and Abdomen. Give IVF's and PRBC's if unstable/hypotensive. Stat Surgical Consult for OR.

115. Calcaneus Fracture: Often occurs after a jump from a Height (Lower vertebrae injuries can also occur with these injuries). Diagnosis is on X-ray (Measure Boehler's Angle). Stat Orthopedic Consult Needed for Possible Surgical Repair.

116. Carbon Monoxide Poisoning: Treatment is 100% Oxygen and in some patients, Hyperbaric Oxygen Chamber

117. Name a Dangerous Type of Mushroom Toxin. Amanita Phalloides. What Symptoms can it cause? Mushrooms can cause Nausea, Vomiting, Bloody Diarrhea, Liver Failure, Coagulopathy, Renal Failure. Usually, the Earlier the onset of symptoms, the Worse the Prognosis.

118. What can Syphilis cause? Painless Chancre, Cardiovascular Complications, Neurological Complications. What is the Treatment? Penicillin

119. Scromboid Poisoning: Redness, Hives, Vomiting, Diarrhea, Abdominal pain, Palpitations, Headache. Treatment is Antihistamine.

120. Carotid Artery Dissection can present with Headache, Neck pain, Facial pain, Horner syndrome, Symptoms of a Stroke. Management is Anticoagulants (unless contraindicated. Contraindicated in intracranial extension of the dissection).

121. When are Anticoagulants **Contraindicated** in Carotid artery Dissection patients? If there is an Intracranial Extension of the Dissection

122. ANUG = Acute Necrotizing Gingivitis (also known as "Trench Mouth") Mouth Infection. Malodorous. Gums are very red. Management is Irrigate with warm water, give Antibiotics and Provide appointment with the Dentist on the same day.

123. Ciguatera Poisoning: Abdominal Pain, Nausea, Vomiting, Diarrhea, Paresthesias in Mouth region, Having an Odd Sensation when Skin touches a Cold item. Bradycardia, Respiratory Distress. Supportive Treatment (ie Fluids, etc).

124. A Patient Sustained a Trauma to the Neck. On Exam you notice an Expanding Hematoma. What is the Next Step? Immediate Operative Intervention. This is one of the "Hard signs".

125. Why should you always only **slowly** correct Hyponatremia? Because if the correction is too rapid, it can cause Cerebral Pontine Myelinosis!

126. A Patient has a Positive Ultrasound FAST exam after a Trauma. What's the next Step. They Need to go to the OR! Consult Surgery Stat!

127. Tooth fractures (Ellis I = Enamel involved, Ellis II = Dentin involved as well, Ellis III = Pulp also involved). Ellis I and II need Dental follow up Same day or Next day. Ellis III Needs a Dentist Immediately.

128. What can you see on a Hypothermia patient's EKG sometimes? Osborn waves (J waves).

129. Necrotizing Enterocolitis: Abdominal pain, GI bleeding, Vomiting that is often Bilious, Diarrhea. Occurs in Infants. Occurs more often in Premature infants. Diagnosis is at times on X-ray. Management is IVF's, NPO, NG tube, IV Antibiotics and a Stat Surgical Consult for Potential Surgical Intervention.

130. Hantavirus: Spread by Rodents and their Secretions (ie. Urine, Feces). Can Manifest as a Pulmonary Syndrome (Cough, Dyspnea, Fever, Bodyaches) or as a Hemorrhagic Fever with Renal Failure (Fever, Abdominal Pain, Headache, Weakness, Renal Failure). Management is Supportive.

131. Ehrlichiosis: Tick-Borne Infection. It causes Fever, Muscle aches, Weakness, Headache, Nausea, Vomiting, Diarrhea, Rash, Injected Conjunctivae. Labs May show Liver Function Test Elevation, Leukopenia and Thrombocytopenia. Management is Doxycycline.

132. Lyme disease: Tick Borne Disease. Starts with Erythema Migrans (Target like Rash). If not treated with Doxycycline, can progress to other symptoms (ie. Cardiovascular (AV blocks), Neurological (Bell's palsy, Meningitis), Rheumatological (Arthritis). Management: Doxycycline. Can consider Ceftriaxone for more severe complications of Lyme (ie. Neurological and Cardiovascular).

133. Roseola: Consider this in a Child with a High Fever and a Rash but Rule Out the more Concerning causes first, like Meningitis! Management for Roseola is Supportive.

134. Rubella: Lymphadenopathy, Fever, Rash, Headache, Conjunctivits, Rhinorrhea. The Vaccine can prevent this.

135. Munchausen by Proxy: This is when a Parent or Caregiver subjects a Child to Unnecessary Tests/Imaging and Subjects the Child to the Patient Role. The Caregiver may go to the extent of tampering with the results.

136. Child abuse: Anytime you see an injury that is Inconsistent with the Child's Age, Suspect Child Abuse (For Instance, a 2 month old Infant with Bruising over the Body, and the Parent states she rolled off the bed). This must be reported to Child Protective Services. Elder Abuse Must Also Be Reported to the Appropriate Authorities.

137. Achilles Tendon Rupture: Diagnosis: An Audible Pop-like sound may be heard at the Time of the Rupture. You can feel the Rupture of the Achilles when Palpating the Patient's Achilles Tendon. Thompson Test: Patient lays in the Prone position, on his/her stomach. When the Examiner Squeezes the Calf, if there is No Plantar Flexion by the Foot, then the Achilles Tendon is Ruptured. Management is to Splint the Foot and Provide Early Orthopedic Follow Up for Possible Surgical Repair. Complete Rupture needs Surgical Repair.

138. Dacrocystitis: Painful, Erythematous and Swollen over the Region where the Lacrimal Sac region is located. Tearing occurs. Needs IV Antibiotics, Warm Compresses and Admission

139. Bronchiolitis: Rhinorrhea, Trouble Breathing Possible (Retractions, etc.), Wheezing. May be due to RSV. In Premature Infants, Infants under 6 months old, Those with Abnormal Vital Signs, Those with Retractions or Any Respiratory Distress, those without improvement after treatments, those with unreliable follow up, consider admitting since the Risk of Apnea is present in young infants with RSV Bronchiolitis. Management is Oxygen, Can try Albuterol Nebulizer treatment, Suction Nasal Secretions. Can try Racemic Epinephrine.

140. Wolff Parkinson White (WPW) is noted on a Patient's EKG. What is One of the Managements to Consider? Procainamide. WPW is due to an Accessory Pathway. EKG shows Delta wave (Slurred QRS Upstroke), Short PR interval.

141. How do you detect a Posterior wall MI on EKG? ST Depressions in V1, V2, V3 and Tall R waves as well. Check Posterior Leads V7-V9 for ST Elevation

142. What are Contraindications to Fibrinolysis in STEMI? Bleeding, Hx of ICH, Aortic Dissection, CVA, Brain Cancer or Mets, Brain lesions, Head Trauma, GI Bleeding

143. What is the Best Management for a STEMI? PCI

144. Jones Fracture: Fracture of the Fifth Metatarsal. There are Complications that can occur if Jones Fractures are not addressed, including Nonunion. Needs Stat Orthopedic Consult. If Displaced, Needs Operative Intervention. If Nondisplaced, Splint, Nonweightbearing, Orthopedic Follow Up on the same day as this Patient may still need Surgical Intervention.

145. What is the Best Treatment for AMS, HAPE and HACE? Descent!

146. What is Often needed for a Circumferential Burn? Escharotomy

147. Infantile Botulism: Poor Feeding, Cry is Weak in Tone, Difficulty Passing Stool, Weakness. Needs Antitoxin and Admit.

148. A Closed Fist Injury: A Punch to the Face leading to a Bite Wound on the Joints of the Metacarpals. Needs a Stat Hand Surgeon/Orthopedic Consult and IV Antibiotics

149. What are Dystonias and How to they present? How do you treat dystonias? Due to cholinergic excess, dystonias may manifest with eyes rolling backwards (opisthotonos), torticollis, back arching backwards, tongue protruding outward in circular motions). Benadryl or Benzotropine are used in the treatment because have Anticholinergic activity

150. A Child Swallowed a Button Battery that is lodged in the Esophagus. What is the Next Step? Stat GI consult for Endoscopic Removal. Button Batteries are Dangerous. Other Reasons for Immediate Endoscopy to Remove a Foreign Body, include Long objects or Sharp objects or Wide Objects or Button Batteries or Complication (ie Perforated Viscous) or Many Foreign Bodies or a Foreign body that is Not Progressing Along.

151. In a patient with Sickle Cell Anemia, who presents with a Stroke or Priapism what Management Measures are Needed? Exchange Transfusion

152. Myasthenia Gravis is a Neuromuscular Disorder that presents with Eye Complaints and can manifest with Respiratory Distress. Weakness of Facial Muscles, Difficulty Swallowing, Ptosis, Diplopia are all Possible Symptoms.

Management is Treatment with Acetylcholinesterase Inhibitors (ie. Pyridostigmine) and Airway Management.

153. What is the Management of Uncomplicated Impetigo (yellow crusted lesions)? Topical Mupirocin. What if it is Complicated? Antibiotics PO.

154. What are the Main Management Principles of Epiglottitis and Retropharyngeal Abscess? Airway Management, ENT Consult Stat, IV Antibiotics

155. Transient Synovitis: Hip pain in children. Can present with Hip pain, Knee pain, Thigh Pain or Limp. Ensure that the patient does not have Septic Arthritis! If the patient surely doesn't have septic arthritis (ie. Negative Arthrocentesis, No clinical findings, No lab findings, Afebrile, Well Appearing), then the Management for Transient Synovitis is No weight-bearing, Orthopedic follow up very soon and supportive measures. If any suspicion for Septic Arthritis, Arthrocentesis, Antibiotics, Admission, Stat Orthopedic Consultation

156. When Correcting DKA in a Pediatric Patient with Fluids, Insulin, etc., if there is too rapid a correction attempted with fluids, what is the detrimental consequence of this? Cerebral Edema.

157. A Child is Not moving his/her arm. You suspect Nursemaid's Elbow. How can you manage this? Get an X-ray to ensure No trauma/Fracture. Then to Reduce the Nursemaid's Elbow, either Supinate and Flex the Forearm or Hyperpronate it. Within minutes, the child will be using the Forearm again.

158. Malignant Otitis Externa: Seen in Diabetics or Elderly Patients with Pain in the Ear. The Exam shows Visualizable Granulation Tissue. Needs Admission for IV Antibiotics and Possible Debridement by the Surgical Specialist/ENT.

159. Legg Calve Perthes: Occurs in Children. Can Manifest with Hip pain, Limp, Knee Pain or Thigh Pain. Due to Avascular Necrosis of the Head of the Femur. Difficulty walking. Diagnosis is X-ray. Management is Stat Orthopedic Consultation and Admission.

160. TMJ Dislocation: The TMJ gets Dislocated. Management is to Cover the Thumbs with Cloth or Gauze and then Place Thumbs on the Back of the Lower Teeth and Push the Jaw Downward and Posteriorly in Direction, to Reduce it. Needs ENT consult/follow-up

161. What is Allowed and What is Contraindicated in Cocaine induced Chest Pain? Aspirin and Benzodiazepines are allowed. However, Beta-Blockers are Contraindicated because they lead to Unopposed Alpha Activity!

162. How can Retinal Detachment present? What is the Diagnosis? What is the Management? It can present as Floaters in the Eyes. It can present with a Sensation of a Curtain Closing over the Eye. The Diagnosis is an Eye Exam with an Opthalmoscope, Ultrasound of the Orbit and the Management is Stat Ophthalmology Consultation. Admit.

163. In a Patient who comes in with Chemical Exposure to the Eyes, What is the Main Management Principle? Irrigate the Eyes with Normal Saline that is Sterile (Can use Morgan Lens).

164. CRAO: Visual Loss. Painless. Due to an Embolus. Needs Ophthalmology Consult Stat. The Management has been to Massage the Globe lightly to attempt to dislodge the clot

165. CRVO: Visual Loss. Painless. See Retinal Hemorrhage on Examination of the Eye. Consult Ophthalmology

166. Le Fort Fractures: Fractures of the Face (See Above Text section). Needs Stat Surgical/ENT Evaluation, IV Antibiotics and Airway Management.

167. A Patient has Vesicles on the Tip of his Nose. His Slit lamp Exam shows a Dendritic like Pattern. What is the Condition and what is the Management? Herpes Zoster Ophthalmicus and the Treatment is Acyclovir or Valacyclovir PO. Also give Antibiotic Eye Drops. Needs Stat Ophthalmology Consultation. Note: When the tip of the nose is involved, always check for Eye involvement.

168. Alcoholic Ketoacidosis: Presents with an Elevated Anion Gap Acidosis and Ketonemia. Patient has a Normal or Low Glucose Level mostly and a Normal or Low Alcohol Level mostly. Management is Thiamine, Dextrose with Normal Saline

169. The Drug, PCP, can cause Violent Behavior and Nystagmus

170. A Patient has Ascending Weakness, starting at Lower Extremities. On Exam, you notice Absent Reflexes. What do you think is going on? Guillain Barre Syndrome.

171. What is the Best Management Modality in a Patient with a STEMI? PCI

172. What does Organophosphate Poisoning Manifest as and What is the Management? Salivation, Vomiting, Diarrhea, Rhinorrhea, Increased Secretions, Weakness. Management is Atropine and Pralidoxime

173. In Patients with Carbon Monoxide Poisoning, which patients get Hyperbaric Oxygen Chamber Treatment? Cardiovascular Symptoms (ie. Myocardial infarction), Neurological symptoms (ie. AMS, Seizure), Any patient with a level >25%, Pregnant patients with a level >15%, Anyone without any improvement on 100% Oxygen Therapy

174. Lisfranc's Fracture: Do a Thorough Neurovascular Exam and Consult Orthopedics Stat for ORIF or Closed Reduction.

175. In an Alcoholic who presents to your ER, who is Altered, Always do a Full Physical Examination, get Lab Work and do a CT Head to ensure that there are No Missed Injuries (like an Intracranial Hemorrhage).

176. A Patient who wants to leave Against Medical Advice (AMA) must be Competent, able to make good judgment, have good insight, must have the Capacity to make good decisions and must understand the full risks of leaving (ie. death, multiorgan failure, disability, etc). Reminder: There are some patients who **cannot** leave Against Medical Advice. For instance, a patient who is Intoxicated **cannot** leave AMA!

177. A Patient Overdosed on Amitriptyline (TCA). What is the Management for a Wide Complex Dysrhythmia? Sodium Bicarbonate. If this same Patient had a Seizure, what would you give? A Benzodiazepine (Lorazepam).

178. How can a Fat Embolism present? Neurological Symptoms (ie. Seizure, AMS, etc.), Petechiae, Respiratory Distress (Chest Pain, Shortness of Breath). Management: Supportive Management (Oxygen, Airway Management, Steroids). What can predispose to a Fat Embolism? Long Bone Fractures.

179. A Patient who is Pregnant and has Vaginal Bleeding and is Rh Negative, needs Rhogam, if she was never given it before.

180. A Patient presents Hypoglycemia Secondary to Sulfonylurea Use. What should be the Management and the Disposition? Give Octreotide, Frequently Monitor Blood Glucose Level and Admit. Why? Must Admit because these patients are prone to Rebound Hypoglycemia, given the Prolonged Action of the Sulfonylurea. For Moderate to Long Acting Insulin Medications Note that these Patients also need Admission for the same reason.

181. Diverticulitis: Can present with LLQ pain, diarrhea. Needs a CT scan Abdomen/ Pelvis. Management: Antibiotics (Ciprofloxacin and Flagyl). Admit if any Complications (ie Abscess, Perforation), Intractable Pain, Nausea/Vomiting, Failed outpatient treatment, unreliable follow up.

182. A patient presents with a Tremor, Anxiety, Fever, Nausea, Vomiting and an Altered Mental Status, Proptosis. What is One of your concerns and What is the Management of this Condition? Thyroid Storm. Give Propranolol, PTU or Methimazole. Then Wait One hour and give Iodide. Give Dexamethasone. Where should this patient get admitted? The ICU.

183. What do you do with a Posterior Hip Dislocation? It needs Immediate Reduction! Otherwise it leads to Avascular Necrosis of the Head of the Femur! Always check the Neurovascular status both before and after the reduction. How do Posterior Hip Dislocations Present? Adducted, Shortened and Internally Rotated

184. A Finger that is Amputated Needs what Management? Irrigate amputated portion. Put the Amputated Finger in a Sterile Gauze Soaked with Saline and Place that in a Plastic Bag. Then place that Bag in Ice Water. But **Don't** let the actual amputated digit touch any ice! Remember it is in a soaked sterile gauze, that is in a plastic bag and the bag is what should be touching the ice water.

185. Brugada Syndrome: Shows a Hunchback looking ST elevation that are in any two leads between V1 to V3. Causes an Incomplete RBBB in appearance. The T wave is inverted. These patients are at risk of suddenly dying. Always think of this in a patient with a Syncopal Episode. Always ask for a Family Cardiac History as it is often Positive. Admit. Cardiology Consult. Management is AICD.

186. What does DKA Manifest as and what is the Management of DKA? Abdominal pain, Nausea, Vomiting, "Kussmauls Respirations" Possible. Presents with Glucose > 250, Acidosis (Low pH, Low Bicarbonate). Elevated Anion Gap. Presence of Ketones (Ketonuria, Ketonemia). Management: IV Fluids (Normal Saline initially and then once the Glucose falls under 250, switch to D5 1/2 NS), Insulin. Need to Close the Anion Gap. Correct the Electrolytes appropriately. Get Hourly FSG, Electrolytes/Metabolic Panel and ABG. Treat the Underlying Cause (ie. Infection). ICU Admission.

187. What Must you think of in a Patient who you believe is Septic who is Not improving with IV fluids? Always keep Adrenal Crisis in mind when managing these patients. These patients should receive Steroids, if Adrenal Crisis is suspected.

188. What is the Management of Ethylene Glycol and Methanol Poisoning? Fomepizole

189. A Patient with Eye Pain, Erythema, and Swelling. Ophthalmoplegia is present. What's the most likely Diagnosis and What's the Diagnostic Study? Orbital Cellulitis. CT Orbit. What is Next? IV Antibiotics, Stat Ophthalmology Consult and Admission

190. A Patient has Abdominal Pain, Nausea, Vomiting and a Hernia that is Strangulated. What should you do? Give IV Antibiotics and Get a Stat Surgery Consultation for Repair in the OR.

191. A Patient presents after Eye Trauma. The Eyeballs are looking Upward Constantly. What is the diagnosis? Orbital Blowout fracture.

192. A Child is Itching her Anus Primarily at Night. What do you think this is and what is the Diagnosis and Treatment? Enterobiasis can cause these symptoms. It is due to Pinworms. Conduct a Scotch Tape Test and Empirically Treat with Albendazole.

193. Central Cord Syndrome: Affects the Upper Extremities more with Weakness. Often the injury is secondary to hyperextension. May affect control of the bladder.

194. Anterior Cord Syndrome: Loss of Pain and Temperature Sensation below the lesion and it also affects the Motor Functioning (Paralysis below the lesion). However, the Vibration/Proprioception Sensation stays intact.

195. Brown Sequard Syndrome: Ipsilateral Loss of Vibration/Proprioception. Ipsilateral Loss of Motor Functioning. Contralateral Loss of Pain and Temperature Sensation.

196. Pain and Temperature Sensation: Spinothalamic Tract.

197. Vibration and Proprioception Sensation: Dorsal Columns

198. Motor Functioning: Corticospinal Tract

199. A Woman has a Sore Throat, Hoarse Voice and Pain in the Ear. Physical exam shows that her Uvula is deviated. What do you think this is and what is the Management? Peritonsillar Abscess and Needs Needle Aspiration, by ENT and Antibiotics.

200. How can Aortic Stenosis Present? Syncope, MI, CHF. What is the Definitive Management that is needed in Symptomatic patients? They need Surgical Aortic Valve Replacement.

201. A Man Dislocated his Knee after a Motor Vehicle Collision. He presents with the Knee Back in place. What should be done and Why? Full Neurological Exam, Full Cardiovascular Exam. Additionally, Needs an Angiography/CT Angiography to ensure that there was No injury to the Popliteal Artery, which is one of the Very

Concerning Complications of a Knee Dislocation. If Present or Suspected based on Clinical Signs, Needs Vascular Surgery Consult Stat.

202. What is Needed in a Patient with Ludwig's Angina? Airway Management and IV Antibiotics. Consult ENT immediately.

203. What is the Management of Necrotizing Fasciitis? IV Antibiotics, Stat Surgery Consult for Surgical Debridement

204. You see Abdominal Contents located in the Chest cavity on a Chest X-ray in a trauma patient. What is your suspected diagnosis and what is the Management? Diaphragmatic Injury and Needs Stat Surgery Consult for Surgical Repair in the OR

205. What is the most likely Management of a Supracondylar Fracture that is Unstable and Displaced? A Thorough Neurovascular Exam, Stat Orthopedic Consult for Operative Intervention, Admission, Further Monitoring

206. What should you always consider in a STEMI patient? Does this patient have an Aortic Dissection? What Medications Would be **Contraindicated** in these Patients? **Contraindicated:** Anticoagulants, Aspirin, Plavix, Thrombolytics are all **Contraindicated** in patients with Dissection. An Aortic Dissection needs Blood Pressure control if the patient is Hypertensive, starting with a Beta Blocker and then Nitroprusside. Patient Needs a Stat Vascular Surgery Consult for Operative Repair.

207. A Patient Presents with Severe Abdominal Pain but the Physical Exam is benign. What should you consider? Mesenteric Ischemia.

208. What Causes High Output Cardiac Failure? Pregnancy, Hyperthyroidism, Anemia that is very severe

209. What do you expect to see on an EKG of a Left Bundle Branch Block (LBBB)? A Wide QRS, A Broad R wave in V5, V6 and a Deep S wave in V1, V2

210. What might you see in a Patient with Globe Rupture? Positive Siedel Sign and A "Teardrop Pupil"

211. What are the Complications of a Hyphema? Acute Narrow Angle Glaucoma and Rebleeding. What do you have to Rule out in a Hyphema? A Globe Rupture. Who do you consult? Stat Ophthalmology Consult.

212. If the Globe is Ruptured, Do **Not** place any pressure on the eye. A Globe Rupture Needs a Stat Ophthalmology Consult to go to the OR. Start IV Antibiotics, Give a Tetanus Shot.

213. Multiple family members present with the same symptoms: Weakness and a Headache. It is February and you are in Canada. What could this be? Carbon Monoxide Poisoning

214. A Patient presents with Back Pain and Leg Weakness. On Physical Examination you notice Saddle Anesthesia, Diminished Rectal Tone and Abnormalities in his Bowel/Bladder Functioning. What is your concern? Cauda Equina Syndrome. What's the Next Step? Stat MRI, Stat Neurosurgery Consultation. Start IV Steroids to Reduce Edema.

215. A Patient with Back Pain and Leg Weakness. The BP is Elevated and the CXR shows a Widened Mediastinum. What should you consider in your Differential Diagnosis that is most likely? Aortic Dissection.

216. Urinary Retention is the One of the Most Sensitive Findings for Cauda Equina Syndrome. May Measure Post Void Residual Volume (<100). You may also find Saddle Anesthesia, Diminished/Loss of Rectal Tone

217. Multifocal Atrial Tachycardia: Often occurs in COPD patients. Presents with Tachycardia, an Irregular Rhythm and on EKG you find at least three different types of P waves. You manage this by treating the precipitating etiology.

218. What medication should you **Not** give children when they have viral syndrome/the flu and Why? Aspirin should **Not** be given because it can cause Reye's Syndrome and in children, it can manifest with Liver Damage, Altered Mental Status, Encephalopathy, Coma

219. What are three ways symptomatic Aortic Stenosis can manifest that can shorten one's survival prognosis? Angina, CHF, Syncope

220. A Patient has Rebound, Guarding on Abdominal Examination. His CXR shows Free Air Under the Diaphragm. What is your Next Step. Stat Surgery Consult for OR. NPO. IV Antibiotics.

221. What EKG finding may you see on a Hypokalemic patient's EKG? U waves, Flattened or Inverted T wave

222. Why should you correct Hyponatremia slowly? To prevent Cerebral Pontine Myelinosis

223. Refrain from providing Medical advice over the Telephone, unless it is to be Evaluated by a Physician/in the ER as soon as possible, as this can have strong legal implications.

224. A Child with DKA has been corrected with fluids too rapidly and presents with weakness, headache and a seizure. What is your biggest concern? Cerebral Edema from rapid fluid correction in this patient. Management needs Mannitol. Elevate the Head of the Bed. Must Decrease the Rate of Fluid because this is the likely precipitant!

225. What Pediatric Patients are at Risk of a UTI? Females <2 years old. Uncircumcised Males < 1 year old. Circumcised Males <6 months old. Any Pediatric Patient with any abnormalities in the Genitourinary System.

226. What is always the most important Management Principle to consider from the start? ABC's! Airway, Breathing, Circulation

First and foremost, if possible, choose a geographic location where you will be happy (Family, Friends, Work environment, Cost of living, Quality of life, Medicolegal environment, etc are only a few factors to take into consideration)

1. What's the **Annual Census** at each of the sites?

2. What is the Type of **Setting** (Academic vs. Community? A bit of Both?

3. Additional Opportunities and Responsibilities (Teaching Medical students at an Affiliated Medical School, Teaching Residents, etc.)

4. Roles in Hospital Committees?

5. **Hours** considered Full time? Part time? Per Diem?

6. Physician **Coverage Hours?** PA/NP Coverage Hours? Scribe coverage Hours? Nurse Coverage Hours? Technician Coverage hours?

7. **Independent Contractor** Status or **Employee** status with **Benefits?**

8. **If Employee Status, What Benefits? Health, Vision, Dental?** (Who pays and How much?) **Retirement? 401K? Matching?** How much? **Disability? Life? Pension?** (Does Employer contribute? Vesting period? When does it Begin?) Partnership? Vesting Period? When does it Begin?

9. **Paid Vacation/Time off?** How many weeks?

10. **CME?** How much?

11. **Malpractice Insurance** included? What type? **Occurrence** (Occurrence is best) or Claims (If Claims Based Policy, Ensure that the Employer Covers the Tail and Not you. It should be, Claims based with tail covered by the Employer, also known as **"Claims with tail covered"**)

12. Is there a Tech present 24/7 for **US? CT? MRI?** (In-house 24/7 or Come in when called, after hours?)

13. Are there **Radiology Readings** 24/7? for X-rays as well (overnight)? Do ER Physicians do Preliminary Readings? X-rays, CT scans, etc.

14. **Compensation?** (Base salary or Hourly rate vs. **Base salary** or **Hourly rate plus RVU**, vs. RVU only)

15. Student Loan **Reimbursement?** Sign on/Relocation/Retention **Bonus?**

16. Any **Malpractice Lawsuits** the hospital is dealing with?

17. Do Doctors cover Adult/Pediatric **Codes on the floor?** Do they do **Procedures on the floor?** Do they cover Floor/ICU for Emergencies?

18. **Ancillary staff** (Nurses, Techs and Hours of coverage, Roles); **Physician Coverage** times, **NP/PA coverage** times? **Scribe** coverage times? Level of experience of staff, Board certified ER doctors?

19. Is there a **High Turnover** for staff? Why?

20. What **Specialty Services** are present? What specialty services are **not** present? What gets transferred out? A few examples of Specialty Services: OBGYN, Cardiothoracic Surgery, Pediatrics, Surgery, Neurosurgery, Neurology, Ophthalmology, ENT, Cardiology, GI, Orthopedics

21. How long does **Credentialing** take?

22. Can I **Shadow** before I start to see how the department runs?

23. Note: if it is a medical director role, is the medical director covered by the malpractice insurance and is additional insurance provided, specific to medical directors? What kind? Does it cover the Medical Directors Role, since many Ordinary Physician Malpractice Insurances do not cover since a portion of the Medical Directors role is outside of the clinical realm?

24. Understand the Pros and Cons of *Employee status* vs. *Independent contractor*

25. *Employee* **Pros**: Health, Vision, Dental Benefits, CME, Paid Vacation, 401K... Possible Matching. Possible Pension. Only pay employee share of FICA while employer pays other portion

26. *Employee Cons*: May have a Lower Hourly rate/Salary because getting benefits, Cannot put as much into 401K (at present, 18,000)

27. *Independent Contractor Cons: N*o benefits, No paid time off, Higher FICA taxes (Pay both portions of FICA tax)

28. *Independent Contractor Pros:* can claim many more work related deductions for business expenses (ie. if car used for business purposes, fuel used for work, educational etc.) and can put much more into 401K (at present, 46,000)

29. Look at the Contract and have an Attorney review it for you.

30. **Term of contract** (1 year, 2 years, etc.) - How long does the contract last?

31. **Restrictive covenants:** If you leave the practice or are asked to leave, how many places and within what radius, what regions/areas are you forbidden from practicing and for how long?

32. **Salary** - Is it what was agreed upon? Is it negotiable?

33. **Termination** - Both parties should have the right to terminate the agreement with a decent amount of time to find a new position or find a replacement (standard is 1 to 3 months); there shouldn't be a clause allowing the employee/IC to be fired without much notice (ie 10 days)...if there is try to negotiate it out of the contract

34. **Scheduling** (equitable days, nights, weekends, holidays?)

35. Does the ER doctor write **Admitting orders/bridging orders?**

36. Are there **Hospitalists** or do patients get admitted to private physicians? If private, is it hard to admit?

37. Take note of the **Turnover rate** - is there a particular reason why it may be high, if it is?

38. Is there good **Camaraderie** between the staff (physicians, nurses, techs, etc.)

39. **Partnership** Opportunities? Is there a Buy-In? How much is the **Buy-in?** Number of Partners?

40. **Contact Information** for Others in the Group or who may have left the Group

I wish you all the best on the written oral board examination, the oral board examination and in your residency/practice/career/future endeavors

References

1. Marx JA, Hockberger RS, Walls RM, et al., 8th ed. Rosen's Emergency Medicine: Concepts and Clinical Practice. Philadelphia, PA: Mosby/Elsevier; 2014. pp. 1-2505.

2. Tintinalli JE, Stapczynski JS, Cline DM, Ma OJ, Cydulka RK, Meckler GD, 7th ed. Tintinalli's Emergency Medicine: A Comprehensive Study Guide. New York, NY: McGraw Hill; 2011. pp. 1-1937.

3. Counselman F, et al; 2013 EM Model Review Task Force: The 2013 Model of Clinical Practice of Emergency Medicine. *Acad Emerg Med* 2014; 1-46.

INDEX

II. Section II: Topics by System

- Hernia
- Boerhaave's
- Caustics (Acids, Alkali)
- Infectious Esophagitis
- GERD
- Pill induced Esophagitis
- Tracheoesophageal Fistula
- Zenker's Diverticulum
- Schatzki Ring, Esophageal stricture
- Scleroderma
- Achalasia
- DES
- Esophageal Foreign Body
- Mallory Weiss Syndrome
- Esophageal Varices
- Cirrhosis
- Hepatic Encephalopathy
- Hepatorenal Failure
- Hepatic Abscess
- Hepatitis
- Biliary Colic
- Cholecystitis
- Calculous Cholecystitis
- Emphysematous Cholecystitis
- Choledocholithiasis
- Cholangitis
- Pancreatitis
- Spontaneous Bacterial Peritonitis
- PUD
- Pyloric Stenosis
- Foreign body in stomach
- Gastritis
- Crohn's
- Small Bowel Obstruction
- Paralytic Ileus
- Aortoenteric Fistula
- Meckel's Diverticulum
- Mesenteric Ischemia
- Ulcerative Colitis
- Appendicitis
- Necrotizing Enterocolitis
- Radiation Colitis
- Hirschprung's Disease
- Large Bowel Obstruction
- Diverticulitis
- Intussusception
- Volvulus
- Perianal Abscess
- Perirectal Abscess
- Pilonidal cyst and abscess
- Proctitis

- Anal Fissure
- Anal fistula
- Foreign Body (Rectal)
- Hemorrhoids
- Rectal Prolapse

ii. Cardiology
- PEA
- SUID
- AAA
- Aortic dissection
- Arterial Thromboembolism
  - Acute Limb Ischemia
- DVT
- PE
- Bradycardia
- SVT
- V-tach
- V-fib
- Torsades
- A-fib, A flutter
- WPW
- Brugada
- Prolonged QT
- AV Blocks
- Hypertrophic Cardiomyopathy
- CHF
- Unstable Angina
- NSTEMI
- STEMI
- Pericardial Tamponade
- Pericarditis
- Endocarditis
- Aortic Stenosis
- Mitral Regurgitation
- Aortic Regurgitation
- Mitral Stenosis
- Hypertensive Emergencies
- LBBB
- RBBB

iii. Dermatology
- Erythema Multiforme
- Erythema Nodosum
- Henoch Schonlein Purpura
- Pityriasis Rosea
- Urticaria
- Pemphigus Vulgaris
- Bullous Pemphigoid
- SJS
- TEN
- Toxic shock syndrome
- Staphylococcal Scalded Skin Syndrome
- Decubitus Ulcer

- Abscess
- Cellulitis
- Erysipelas
- Scarlet Fever
- Impetigo
- Necrotizing Fascisti
- Herpes Simplex
- Herpes Zoster
- Scabies
- Rocky Mountain Spotted Fever
- Rubella
- Measles
- Erythema Infectiosum
- Molluscum Contagiosum
- Atopic dermatitis
- Contact dermatitis
- Psoriasis
- Tines infection
- Basal cell carcinoma
- Kaposi's Sarcoma
- Melanoma
- Squamous cell carcinoma

iv. Endocrine, Metabolic
- Adrenal Crisis
- Cushing's Syndrome
- Hypercalcemia
- Hypocalcemia
- Hypokalemia
- Hyperkalemia
- Hyponatremia
- Hypernatremia
- Hypermagnesemia
- Hypomagnesemia
- Hypophosphatemia
- Hyperphosphatemia
- Diabetes
- HHS
- DKA
- Hypoglycemia
- Wernicke-Korsakoff
- Hyperthyroidism
- Thyroid Storm
- Apathetic Hyperthyroidism
- Hypothyroidism
- Myxedema Coma
- Metabolic Acidosis
- Pheochromocytoma

v. Environment
- Bee sting
- Black widow spider bite
- Brown recluse spider bite
- Animal bite

- Cat bite
- Human bite
- Dog bite
- Jellyfish sting
- Stingray
- Coral snake
- Rattlesnake (Viperidae)
- Dysbarism
- Barotrauma
- Air Gas Embolism
- Decompression Syndrome
- Lightning Strike
- Acute Mountain Sickness
- HACE
- HAPE
- Submersion Incidents
- Heat Exhaustion
- Heat Stroke
- Frostbite
- Hypothermia
- Radiation Emergencies

vi. Head, Eye, Ear, Nose, Throat   *80-85*
- Foreign body (Ear)
- Labyrinthitis
- Mastoiditis
- Meniere's disease
- Otitis media
- Otitis externa
- Malignant otitis externa
- Perforated TM
- Corneal Abrasion
- Corneal Ulcer
- Enophthalmitis
- Chalazion
- Hordeolum
- Acute narrow angle glaucoma
- hyphen
- Hypopyon
- Retrobulbar hematoma
- Iritis
- Retinal detachment
- CRAO
- CRVO
- Periorbital cellulitis
- Orbital cellulitis
- Blepharitis
- Conjunctivitis
- Dacrocystitis
- Chemical burn to the eye
- Eye foreign body
- Optic neuritis
- Cavernous sinus thrombosis
- Epistaxis

- Nose foreign body
- Sinusitis
- Nasal fracture
- Ludwig's Angina
- Sialolithiasis
- Epiglottitis
- Tracheitis
- Peritonsillar Abscess
- Pharyngitis
- Infectious Mononucleosis
- Retropharyngeal Abscess

vii. Hematology/Oncology
- Blood transfusion
- Hemophilia A
- DIC
- Thrombocytopenia
- HIT
- ITP
- VWD
- HUS, TTP
- Sickle cell anemia
- Iron deficiency
- Hemolytic anemia
- Aplastic anemia
- Megaloblastic anemia
- Methemoglobinemia
- Leukemia
- Multiple Myeloma
- Leukopenia
- Hodgkin lymphoma
- Non-hodgkin lymphoma
- Neutropenic fever
- Tumor lysis syndrome
- SVC Syndrome
- Hypercalcemia

viii. Immunology
- Reiter's
- Raynaud's
- Scleroderma
- Rheumatoid Arthritis
- SLE
- Temporal arteritis
- Takayasu arteritis
- Allergic reaction
- Anaphylaxis
- Angioedema
- Transplant related problems
- Kawasaki syndrome
- Rheumatic Fever
- Sarcoidosis
- Post-streptococcal Glomerulonephritis

- Meningitis
- Guillain Barre
- Myasthenia Gravis
- Parkinson's disease
- Pseudotumor Cerebri
- Febrile seizure
- Seizure in a VP Shunt patient
- Neonatal seizure
- Status Epilepticus
- Spinal cord compression
- ICH
- SAH
- Ischemic CVA
- TIA

xii. Obstetrics and Gynecology
- PID
- Fitz Hugh Curtis
- TOA
- Ovarian torsion
- Bartholin's abscess
- Foreign body
- Vaginitis
- Candidiasis
- Trichomoniasis
- Abortion
  - Threatened, Missed, Incomplete, Inevitable, Complete, Septic
- Ectopic Pregnancy
- Heterotopic pregnancy
- Molar pregnancy
- Preeclampsia
- Eclampsia
- HELLP syndrome
- Gestational trophoblastic disease
- Abruptio Placentae
- Placenta Previa
- Hyperemesis Gravidarum
- Premature Labor
- PROM
- Complications of Labor
- Postpartum Complications

xiii. Renal/GU
- ARF
- Complications of Dialysis
- Glomerulonephritis
- Nephrotic syndrome
- Cystitis
- Pyelonephritis
- Balanitis
- Balanoposthitis
- Epididymitis
- Fournier's Gangrene
- Prostatitis

- Urethritis
- Paraphimosis
- Phimosis
- Priapism
- Testicular Torsion
- HUS
- Kidney stone
- Uremic encephalopathy

xiv. Pulmonary
- Croup
- Epiglottitis
- Foreign body (airway)
- Bronchiolitis
- Asthma
- COPD
- Cystic fibrosis
- Pleural effusion
- Pneumomediastinum
- Pneumothorax
- Empyema
- Mediastinhtis
- Pulmonary embolism
- Lung abscess
- Pneumonia
- TB
- Pertussis
- Noncardiogenic pulmonary edema
- Tracheotomy tube complications
- Septic emboli

xv. Toxicology
- Tylenol
- NSAISs
- Salicylates
- Ethylene Glycol
- Methanol
- Anticholinergic
- Cholinergic
- Anticoagulants
- TCA
- Serotonin Syndrome
- Neuroleptic Malignant Syndrome
- Carbon Monoxide
- Digitalis
- Beta blocker
- Calcium channel blocker
- Cocaine
- Cyanide
- Hydrogen sulfide
- Hypoglycemic/Insulin
- Iron
- Marine toxins
- Methemoglobinemia
- Mushroom

- Organophosphate
- Opioids
- Sympathomimetics
- Chemical warfare agents
- Scromboid poisoning
- Hydrogen Fluoride
- Lithium
- Strychnine
- Arsenic
- Isopropanolol
- Ciguatera

- ABC's
- Abdominal trauma
- Chest trauma
- Burn
- Bite wound
- High pressure injection wound
- Amputated digit
- Head/Face Trauma
- C-spine trauma
- GU Trauma
- Neck trauma
- Salter Harris Fractures (Pediatric)
- Nursemaid's elbow
- Pelvis fracture
- Extremity Trauma
- Multisystem Trauma

III. Section III: Oral Board Review

- *Beta blocker overdose*
- *TCA overdose*
- *Aortic Dissection*
- *AAA*
- *Brugada's Syndrome*
- *Wellen's Syndrome*
- *STEMI*
- *STEMI (Anterior)*
- *STEMI (Inferior)*
- *STEMI (Posterior)*
- *Pulmonary Embolism*
- *Simple Pneumothorax*
- *Cardiac Tamponade*
- *DVT*
- *Tension pneumothorax*
- *Necrotizing Fasciitis*
- *Ovarian Torsion*
- *PID*
- *TOA*
- *Ectopic Pregnancy*
- *Meningitis*

- Eclampsia
- Subarachnoid Hemorrhage
- Ventricular Tachycardia
- CVA
- Renal Colic
- Pericarditis
- Child Abuse
- Alcohol Withdrawal
- Carotid Artery Dissection
- Vertebral Artery Dissection
- Cavernous Sinus Thrombosis
- Heat Stroke
- Mesenteric Ischemia
- SBO
- Dialysis Patients and Complications
- Hyperkalemia
- Intussusception
- Appendicitis
- Thyroid Storm
- HUS
- TTP
- Hypertensive Emergency
- Status Epilepticus
- Hypoglycemia
- Guillain Barre
- Rocky Mountain Spotted Fever
- Peritonsillar Abscess
- Retropharyngeal Abscess
- Temporal Arteritis
- Septic Arthritis
- Prolonged QT syndrome
- Torsades
- Tylenol Overdose
- Asthma
- Diverticulitis
- Epidural Abscess, Spinal Cord Compression
- Perforated Viscous
- Cholecystitis
- Digoxin Toxicity
- Aspirin Overdose
- Pyelonephritis
- Anaphylaxis
- Vatical Bleed
- Sepsis
- CO Poisoning
- DVT
- Snake Bite
- Cellulitis
- Acute Narrow Angle Glaucoma
- Gout
- Pseudogout
- Septic Arthritis
- Gonococcal Arthritis
- SCFE

- *Pneumonia*
- *Cauda Equina Syndrome*
- *Cardiac Arrest*
- *Sickle Cell Anemia*
- *CHF*
- *Ludwig's Angina*
- *Henoch Schonlein Purpura*
- *Steven Johnson Syndrome*
- *Fournier's Gangrene*
- *Hypoglycemia*
- *DKA*
- *Pyloric Stenosis*
- *Fever in Neonate*
- *Boerhaave's syndrome*
- *Testicular Torsion*
- *Febrile Seizure*
- *Human bite*
- *Cat Bite, Dog Bite*
- *Iron Overdose*
- *Epidural Hematoma*
- *Subdural Hematoma*
- *Kawasaki*
- *Eclampsia*
- *Croup*
- *Chest pain for Cocaine Use*
- *Fever in the Pediatric Patient*
- *Lisfranc fracture*
- *Spontaneous Bacterial Peritonitis*
- *Incarcerated Hernia, Strangulated Hernia*
- *Burn Patient*
- *Myxedema Coma*
- *Adrenal Crisis*
- *ALTE*
- *A few helpful Hints*

IV. <u>Section IV: Rapid Review! Quick Questions & Answers and A Quick Review of Key Concepts to Know!</u>

- **Contains 226 Bullet Points and Questions/Answers to Many of the Main Points in Emergency Medicine!**
- *Cholecystitis*
- *EMTALA*
- *Retrobulbar Hematoma*
- *Fournier's Gangrene*
- *Mesenteric Ischemia*
- *Acute Narrow Angle Glaucoma*
- *TTP*
- *Septic Arthritis*
- *Pseugogout*
- *Gout*
- *Toxic Shock Syndrome*
- *Pseudomonas: Corneal Ulcer in a Contact Lens Wearer and Otitis Externa (Swimmer's Ear)*

- Jellyfish Sting
- Stingray
- Coral Snake Bite
- Anaphylaxis
- Inferior Wall MI, Right Ventricular Infarction
- Posterior Wall MI
- Testicular Torsion
- Aortic Dissection
- Wellen's Syndrome
- Hypertrophic Cardiomyopathy
- CHF
- COPD
- Asthma
- Digoxin Toxicity
- Hyperkalemia
- Complete Heart Block
- Ruptured AAA
- PEA
- Inferior Wall MI
- Scaphoid Fracture
- Appendicitis
- Ectopic Pregnancy
- Aortic Dissection
- Spinal Cord Compression
- Epidural Abscess
- Tension Pneumothorax
- Gas Gangrene
- Cardiac Tamponade
- Croup
- Perforated Viscous
- Torsades
- Ventricular Fibrillation
- Atrial Fibrillation
- Small Bowel Obstruction
- Neonatal Fever
- TCA Overdose
- Subarachnoid Hemorrhage
- Meningitis
- Spontaneous Bacterial Peritonitis
- Cholangitis
- Eclampsia
- Placenta Previa
- Kidney Stone
- Altitude Sickness (AMS, HACE, HAPE)
- SCFE
- Pulmonary Embolism
- Beta blocker overdose
- Calcium channel overdose
- Ruptured Globe
- Esophageal Varices
- Pheochromocytoma
- Endocarditis
- Transplant Complications
- Pancreatitis

- Boerhaave's Syndrome
- TIA
- Rheumatic Fever
- Fournier's Gangrene
- TEN
- HSP
- V-Tach
- Basilar Skull Fracture
- CRAO
- Temporal Arteritis
- DIC
- Adrenal Crisis
- Pregnancy and UTI
- Intussusception
- Kawasaki Disease
- Epiglottitis
- Acute Limb Ischemia
- Delirium Tremens
- Anticholinergic Toxidrome
- Cerebral Venous Thrombosis
- Methemoglobinemia
- Posterior Epistaxis
- Malignant Otitis Externa
- Iron Overdose
- PCP Pneumonia
- Corneal Ulcer
- SVC Syndrome
- Infectious Mononucleosis
- Cavernous Sinus Thrombosis
- Mallet Finger
- High Pressure Injection Injury
- WPW
- Urethral Injury
- Compartment Syndrome
- RMSF
- Auricular Hematoma
- Aortoenteric Fistula
- Serotonin Syndrome
- Neuroleptic Malignant Syndrome
- PID
- Heat Stroke
- Jersey Finger
- Cyanide Poisoning
- Fight Bite
- Flexor Tenosynovitis
- Hyphema
- Tuba-Ovarian Abscess
- Pelvis Fracture
- Calcaneus Fracture
- Carbon Monoxide Poisoning
- Mushroom Toxicity
- Syphilis
- Scromboid Poisoning
- Carotid Artery Dissection

- ANUG
- Ciguatera Poisoning
- Neck Trauma
- Hyponatremia
- US FAST
- Tooth Fractures
- Hypothermia
- Necrotizing Enterocolitis
- Hantavirus
- Ehrlichiosis
- Lyme Disease
- Roseola
- Rubella
- Munchausen by Proxy
- Child Abuse
- Achilles Tendon Rupture
- Dacrocystitis
- Bronchiolitis
- WPW
- Posterior wall MI
- STEMI
- Jones Fracture
- AMS, HACE, HAPE
- Circumferential Burn
- Infantile Botulism
- Closed Fist Injury
- Dystonia
- Button Battery in Esophagus
- Sickle cell anemia
- Myasthenia Gravis
- Impetigo
- Epiglottitis
- Retropharyngeal Abscess
- Transient Synovitis
- DKA
- Nursemaid's Elbow
- Malignant otitis externa
- Legg Calve Perthes
- TMJ Dislocation
- Cocaine induced chest pain
- Retinal Detachment
- Chemical exposure to eyes
- CRAO
- CRVO
- Le Fort Fractures
- Herpes Zoster Opthalmicus
- Alcoholic Ketoacidosis
- Supracondylar Fracture
- Guillain Barre
- STEMI
- Organophosphate Poisoning
- Carbon Monoxide Poisoning
- Lisfranc's fracture
- ICH

- AMA (Administrative)
- TCA Overdose
- Fat embolism
- Rhogam
- Hypoglycemia
- Diverticulitis
- Thyroid Storm
- Posterior Hip dislocation
- Amputated digit
- Brugada Syndrome
- DKA
- Adrenal Crisis
- Ethylene Glycol poisoning
- Orbital Cellulitis
- Hernia
- Orbital Blowout Fracture
- Enterobiasis
- Central Cord Syndrome
- Anterior Cord Syndrome
- Brown Squared Syndrome
- Peritonsillar Abscess
- Aortic Stenosis
- Knee Dislocation
- Ludwig Angina
- Necrotizing Fascisti
- Diaphragm injury
- Supracondylar Fracture
- Aortic Dissection
- Mesenteric Ischemia
- High Output Cardiac Failure
- LBBB
- Globe rupture
- Hyphema
- CO poisoning
- Cauda equina syndrome
- Aortic dissection
- SCC, CES
- Multifocal atrial tachycardia
- Reyes syndrome
- Aortic Stenosis
- Perforated Viscous
- Hypokalemia
- Hyponatremia
- Cerebral Edema from Too Rapid Fluid Correction in a DKA patient
- ABC's